Can't Bend? Can't Snap? Can't Stop Laughing!

Jason M. Aucoin

Jason M. Aucoin

Can't Bend? Can't Snap? Can't Stop Laughing!

Packing Tips, Mental Prep, and All the Weird Stuff Nobody Told You About

Jason M. Aucoin

Packing Tips, Mental Prep, and All the Weird Stuff Nobody Told You About

© 2025 by Jason M. Aucoin

All rights reserved. No part of this publication may be reproduced, distributed, or transmitted in any form or by any means, including photocopying, recording, or other electronic or mechanical methods, without the prior written permission of the publisher, except in the case of brief quotations embodied in critical reviews and certain other noncommercial uses permitted by copyright law.

Jason M. Aucoin

About the book

Can't bend? Can't snap? Cannot Stop Laughing! Tips for packing, mental preparation, and weird stuff you didn't know about

If you've ever been told, "It's just joint surgery, you'll be fine," only to wonder why fine comes with pain meds, grab bars, and an emotional rollercoaster, this book is for you.

This is not your typical clinical guide. It's the road map we all wish we had before surgery day—a combination of practical advice, emotional honesty, hilarious hindsight, and unfiltered wisdom from real patients, professionals, and caregivers.

Why This Book Matters

Because joint surgery is more than just a physical procedure; it is a complete life disruption. While your surgeon may explain the screws and sutures, nobody really walks you through the things that feel equally important:

- How to pack a hospital bag without forgetting the one thing you'll miss the most.
- What to say (and not say) when someone offers to help. How to find meaning in a day when your biggest accomplishment was putting on socks by yourself. Learn why certain post-op gadgets can save your sanity (and others should be donated) and address concerns about pain medication, rest, and healing.

What You Will Gain

Clarity. Confidence. A lot of "Oh thank God, it's not just me."

You'll finish this book with a plan, a laugh, and a fresh perspective. Whether you're having your first or fifth procedure, this guide will assist you:

- Prepare your mind, home, and relationships for surgery and recuperation.
- Maintain resilience through post-op pain, setbacks, and small victories.
- Advocate for yourself with your care team and insurance company.
- Feel seen, supported, and slightly less alone in a journey that is more common than anyone admits.

This is your joint surgery survival kit—honest, hopeful, and just irreverent enough to make you feel like you're walking with a friend the entire time.

Because you can't bend or snap—but with this book? You can keep going. Maybe even laugh about it.

Jason M. Aucoin

TABLE OF CONTENT

Introduction 8

1: UNDERSTANDING YOUR JOINT AND DIAGNOSIS...10

2: QUESTIONS TO ASK YOUR SURGEON...14

3: WHAT TO EXPECT AT YOUR PRE-OP APPOINTMENT...19

4: PREHABILITATION...25

5: MEDS, DIET, & HOME PREP...31

6: THE NIGHT BEFORE...37

7: KNEE SURGERY - PRE & POST BREAKDOWN...44

8: HIP SURGERY - PREP & RECOVERY TIPS...53

9: SHOULDER SURGERY - WHAT YOU NEED TO KNOW...61

10: ELBOW & WRIST SURGERY ESSENTIALS...68

11: ANKLE & FOOT SURGERIES: STEP-BY-STEP RECOVERY...75

12: SPINAL JOINT SURGERIES...81

13: SMALL JOINT SURGERIES: FINGERS & TOES...87

14: JOINT REPLACEMENTS VS. ARTHROSCOPIES...90

15: PEDIATRIC JOINT SURGERY CONSIDERATIONS...96

Packing Tips, Mental Prep, and All the Weird Stuff Nobody Told You About

16: GERIATRIC JOINT SURGERY CONSIDERATIONS...100

17: MULTI-JOINT CONSIDERATIONS AND COMPLEX CASES...104

18: PAIN MANAGEMENT (REAL TALK)...108

19: PHYSICAL THERAPY: LOVE IT OR HATE IT, YOU NEED IT...114

20: COMPLICATIONS TO WATCH FOR...122

21: TOOLS AND GADGETS THAT HELP YOU HEAL SMARTER...131

22: RETURNING TO NORMAL LIFE (OR YOUR NEW NORMAL)...138

About the Author   143

Can't Bend? Can't Snap? Can't Stop Laughing!

Jason M. Aucoin

INTRODUCTION

If you're reading this, you're probably about to have joint surgery or have recently had one and are wondering what happened. Either way, welcome. I am glad you are here.

This book began with a simple realization: No one truly prepares you for what joint surgery is like. The brochures are sterile, the surgeon's explanations are efficient, but the internet is a bit of a horror show. But what's the reality? It's messy, emotional, confusing, funny at times, and profoundly human.

As a medical writer and health journalist, I've covered surgeries, researched protocols, and interviewed some of the most brilliant minds in orthopedics. But it wasn't until I started speaking with real patients—people limping through rehab, icing at 2 a.m., crying in frustration over sock aids and shower chairs—that I realized what was missing: real talk. Not just the details, but the felt experience. The things we don't say aloud in waiting rooms or after surgeries.

So I wrote the book that I wished someone had given me before surgery. A guide who not only tells you what will happen, but also describes how it might feel. One that recognizes the anguish, the fears, the awkward moments—and the small, ridiculous victories that somehow mean everything.

Packing Tips, Mental Prep, and All the Weird Stuff Nobody Told You About

Whether you're dealing with a new hip, a torn ligament, a frozen shoulder, or a fused spine, this book won't sugarcoat or scare you. It is here to provide clarity, laughter, empathy, and practical strategies—things that every patient deserves but rarely gets.

You'll hear from surgeons, therapists, caregivers, and—most importantly—patients like yourself. You'll learn how to prepare (and over prepare), what to expect when expectations fail, and how to reclaim your independence one small, tenacious step at a time.

Because, yes, joint surgery can be overwhelming. But you are not alone. You are a member of a very large, very tough, and very tired club. And, while you may not be able to bend or snap right now, I guarantee that you will laugh again.

This book is for you.

Jason M. Aucoin

PART ONE

PRE-OP PREP FOR ANY JOINT SURGERY

Packing Tips, Mental Prep, and All the Weird Stuff Nobody Told You About

1

UNDERSTANDING YOUR JOINT AND DIAGNOSIS

Or "Why Your Knee is Basically a Moody Mechanical Octopus"

The First Snap, Crackle, and Pop

It usually starts with something simple. A jog that finishes with a wobble. A sharp pain occurred while picking up the dog's bowl. Or, as Dave, a 49-year-old high school basketball coach, described it, a loud pop followed by "a tsunami of regret."

"I thought it was a cramp," Dave explained. "But then my leg gave out. As if it were suddenly on strike."

When something goes wrong in a joint—whether it's the knee, shoulder, or something less glamorous like the ankle—you're thrown into the perplexing world of orthopedic terms, imaging scans, and the fun game of waiting for the specialist to call you back.

But, before you get an MRI and a surgery date, it's important to understand what your joint is, how it broke down, and what your diagnosis actually means.

What Is a Joint, Anyway?

In medical terms, a joint is where two or more bones meet and move against one another. But that makes it sound a lot more relaxed than it is. Joints are biological engineering marvels—complex intersections where bones, cartilage, ligaments, tendons, and fluid all interact (when they feel like it).

Can't Bend? Can't Snap? Can't Stop Laughing!

Jason M. Aucoin

Dr. Melissa Grant, an orthopedic surgeon at Mount Sinai, describes it this way:

> "Your joint is like a band: the bones are the instruments, the cartilage is the soundproofing, the ligaments are the roadies who hold everything together, and the synovial fluid is...well, the coffee. "It keeps things running smoothly."

There are several types of joints:

- Hinge joints (such as knees and elbows) allow you to bend and straighten.
- Ball-and-socket joints (hips and shoulders) are ideal for rotation and full range of motion.
- Gliding joints (wrists, ankles): These allow for small, precise movements.

Each one is vulnerable in unique ways, and depending on your age, activity level, and genetics, yours may decide to betray you sooner than expected.

How Things Go Wrong

Joints are designed for movement, but they don't like surprises. Repetitive strain, sudden impact, aging, inflammation, or even your own immune system can all damage the machinery. The majority of joint problems fall into a few common categories:

1. Injury

Consider torn ACLs, dislocated shoulders, or fractures that penetrate the joint space. You don't have to be an athlete to get them; sometimes simply stepping off a curb at the wrong angle will suffice.

2. Degeneration

This show is centered on arthritis. The cartilage deteriorates, bones rub together, and each step feels as if your skeleton is complaining.

3. Inflammation

Packing Tips, Mental Prep, and All the Weird Stuff Nobody Told You About

Rheumatoid arthritis, gout, and other autoimmune diseases can cause joint inflammation even in the absence of injury or wear and tear.

4. Alignment or structural issues

Your body's natural architecture may predispose you to joint problems. Flat feet, uneven hips, and a misshapen patella (knee cap) can all disrupt the system.

Identifying the Problem

Getting a proper diagnosis is like solving a mystery in which your joint is the untrustworthy narrator. Here's how medical investigations typically go down:

`Step One: The Exam`

Your doctor will bend, twist, and probably ask you to do something painful. This is not sadism; it is how they determine which structures are most likely involved.

`Step Two: Imaging`

- X-rays reveal bone and alignment issues.
- MRIs are VIP passes into soft tissues such as cartilage and ligaments.
- CT scans provide a detailed 3D image that is commonly used for surgical planning.
- Ultrasound is useful for real-time imaging of tendons and fluid pockets.

`Step 3: "The Talk"`

This is when your doctor uses unfamiliar terms like meniscus tear, rotator cuff strain, labral damage, osteoarthritis, and chondromalacia. You are allowed to ask, "Can you say that in English?" Actually, you should.

What Your Diagnosis Does Not Tell You (But You Should Know)

Can't Bend? Can't Snap? Can't Stop Laughing!

Jason M. Aucoin

Most doctors don't tell you this, but the same MRI result can mean very different things to different people.

Dr. Grant explains.

"We've seen 70-year-olds with bad-looking knees on MRI who feel fine, and 30-year-olds with minor wear who are in agony. Diagnosis isn't everything; it's only one part of the puzzle."

So, what matters?

- Your pain and mobility limitations.
- How much the problem interferes with your normal life.
- Your objectives—whether it's walking your dog without limping or running a marathon.

The best treatment—and whether surgery is appropriate for you—depends on all of these factors, not just the scan results.

The more knowledgeable you are, the more effective your conversations with doctors, physical therapists, and even your own fears will be.

What about Dave, our high school coach? He eventually learned he had a torn meniscus and chose arthroscopic surgery. But the real turning point, he told me, wasn't the operation, but rather finally understanding what went wrong and why.

"Once I got the full picture," he said, *"I stopped feeling broken. I began to feel like someone with a plan.*

Packing Tips, Mental Prep, and All the Weird Stuff Nobody Told You About

2
Questions to Ask Your Surgeon

Or: "What to Say When You're Wearing a Paper Gown and Your Brain Goes Blank"

The silence of the scrubs.

When Lani finally sat down with her orthopedic surgeon, she had a list. It was handwritten, folded twice, and placed in her handbag alongside an emergency chocolate bar. She had Googled, contacted her support group, and even called her cousin, a nurse. She had finished her homework.

And then the surgeon walked in—confident, rushed, and polite—and Lani, 58, who had been suffering from crippling knee pain for five years, forgot every question.

"I just nodded," she explained later. "He said things like 'scope' and 'reconstruction,' and I was like, okay, that sounds good. I didn't want to appear dumb."

Why the Right Questions Matter

Surgeons are inherently action-oriented. They want to fix things. Thank goodness for that. But while they're preparing to repair your joint, you're still trying to figure out what's wrong, how they intend to fix it, and what your life might be like afterward.

That is why asking questions is not only logical, but also necessary. You're not just getting ready for surgery; you're looking for someone to open up your body and rearrange your parts. That's a huge deal.

Jason M. Aucoin

Dr. Sonya Levesque, a joint reconstruction specialist, states it bluntly:

"I enjoy informed patients. Ask me the hard questions. If a surgeon becomes annoyed by your questions, it's a red flag."

Real Talk: Why Don't We Ask Enough

Fear. Embarrassment. Trust. Overwhelm. Many people think:

- "The doctor knows best."
- "I don't want to take up too much time."
- "What if I ask a dumb question?"

Remember, this is your body, recovery, and journey. You deserve to know what is going to happen to you—and what your options are.

So let's go over what you should ask before anyone pulls out a scalpel.

Top questions you should (actually) ask your surgeon.

1. What is my diagnosis, and how bad is it?

You need more than just a label. Ask:

* "Can you show me the MRI/X-ray and explain what we're looking at?"
* "What stage is this condition in?"
* "Are there signs of damage elsewhere in the joint?"

2. Do I really need surgery now?

Surgery is not always an urgent matter. However, it is frequently elective or can be avoided with other treatments.

* "What happens if I wait?"
* "What non-surgical options are left?"
* "How long can I delay this safely?"

3. What kind of surgery are we discussing?

Packing Tips, Mental Prep, and All the Weird Stuff Nobody Told You About

You want to know:

* Is this arthroscopic (minimally invasive) or open?
* Are you fixing, removing, or replacing anything?
* "What will you be doing in there, exactly?"

Lani claims that this was her turning point:

"I thought I was going to get a knee replacement. It turned out that it was just a meniscus trim. I had no idea there were levels in this stuff."

4. What are the risks and potential complications?

Do not be afraid to take this on. Ask:

* "What are the most common complications?"
* "What should I be watching for post-op?"
* "What's your complication rate with this procedure?"

This is not rude; it is responsible. A good surgeon will respond confidently.

5. What will recovery look like for someone like me?

This question changes everything. You want real-world expectations rather than textbook answers.

* "How long will I need to use a walker/crutches?"
* "When can I have a shower? Drive? "Go back to work?"
* "What's the typical timeline for pain, swelling, and normal function?"
* And if you're over 60, have other conditions, or aren't particularly active, ask what recovery looks like for someone in your situation.

6. What type of physical therapy will I need, and when should I begin?

Rehabilitation is only half the battle. Make sure you ask:

* "Do you refer to specific PTs or clinics?"

Can't Bend? Can't Snap? Can't Stop Laughing!

- "Will I need in-home therapy at first?"
- "How often and for how long?"

7. How many of these surgeries have you completed?

This is your right. Don't be concerned about sounding challenging.

- "How long have you been doing this specific procedure?"
- "How many do you perform each year?"
- "What outcomes have you seen with patients like me?"

Dr. Levesque notes:

"A good surgeon won't simply rattle off numbers. They'll tell you what they've learned by doing it over and over."

8. Who should I contact if I have questions or problems following surgery?

Surgery is not a one-day event. It is a process. Know who your point person is.

- "Will I get a nurse navigator?"
- "Can I email or call you with concerns?"
- "What's the response time for post-op issues?"

Patient Stories: Questions that Changed Everything

Chris, 42, runs with hip pain.
He almost scheduled a hip replacement—until he inquired about recovery time and was told it could take up to a year.

"That gave me pause." I sought a second opinion and was prescribed a cortisone injection and targeted physical therapy. Surgery is now on the back burner.

Rita, 67, has shoulder arthritis.
Her surgeon did not mention that she would lose some mobility after a full shoulder replacement—until she asked.

"Will I be able to reach my top kitchen shelf?"

Packing Tips, Mental Prep, and All the Weird Stuff Nobody Told You About

It turns out she wouldn't. That altered how she prepared her home and shifted her expectations.

Bonus: Questions you didn't know to ask.

* "Do I need to stop taking supplements or medications before surgery?"
* "Will you be using general anesthesia or regional?"
* "Can I donate my own blood beforehand?"
* "Are there videos or diagrams you recommend I watch?"
* "What should I eat—or avoid—in the weeks leading up to surgery?"

Write it down, bring a buddy, and take notes.

Do not rely on your memory. Take a written list of questions (or this chapter!) to your appointment. Invite a friend or family member to come along and take notes—or at least listen.

Recording the conversation on your phone—with the surgeon's permission—can also help you go over details later, when the nerves have worn off and the questions return.

This is a conversation and not a lecture.

The most significant shift in modern medicine is that patients are no longer passive. You aren't just lying on the table. You are taking an active role in your healing. You're establishing a relationship with the person wielding the scalpel.

As Lani told me weeks after her surgery:

"Once I began asking the right questions, I stopped feeling like a body on a conveyor belt. I felt like a human being in control of her decisions."

Jason M. Aucoin

3
WHAT TO EXPECT AT YOUR PRE-OP APPOINTMENT

Or, "Congratulations! You're Officially a Science Project"

The Countdown Begins

It's real now. The decision has been made, the surgery date circled on your calendar (in ink), and suddenly, you find yourself at the pre-operative appointment—a deceptively routine-sounding checkpoint that is actually a jam-packed, emotionally loaded gateway to your operation.

As one patient, Carla, 63, said to me:

"It felt like airport security for my body. Blood pressure here, medical history there, and a hundred questions later, I'm just hoping they let me on the plane."

And she's not wrong. This appointment is designed to clear you for surgery, flag any risks, and prep your body and brain for what's coming. But it can also be overwhelming, technical, and full of jargon. So let's break it down, step by step, so you know exactly what's coming—and how to walk in feeling confident, not clueless.

What Is a Pre-Op Appointment, Really?

Think of this as your surgical passport office. It's where your medical team gathers the Intel they need to:

- Assess your current health
- Minimize surgical risks
- Optimize your body for healing

Packing Tips, Mental Prep, and All the Weird Stuff Nobody Told You About

- Prepare you mentally and logistically for surgery day and beyond

It usually takes place 1–4 weeks before your operation, either at the surgeon's office, a hospital-based pre-op clinic, or virtually, depending on your health system and procedure.

What Happens at the Pre-Op Appointment?

It varies a little depending on the joint you're getting repaired or replaced, your overall health, and your facility. But here's the core itinerary:

1. Medical History Review

* Be ready to talk about your entire life, from chickenpox to cholesterol.
* All medical conditions (past and present)
* Surgeries you've had
* Family history of heart disease, anesthesia reactions, or bleeding disorders
* Medications, supplements, vitamins, herbal remedies (yes, even that ginseng tea)
* Allergies (especially to medications, latex, or anesthesia)

TIP: Bring a written list. Your surgeon will love you for it.

2. Physical Exam

Expect a once-over that may include:

* Listening to your heart and lungs
* Taking your blood pressure, pulse, weight, and oxygen levels
* Checking the joint in question for range of motion, swelling, and strength

They're not just confirming you're human. They're looking for red flags that could delay or complicate surgery—like uncontrolled hypertension, infection, or undiagnosed sleep apnea.

3. Pre-Surgical Testing

Depending on your age and health:

* Blood tests (to check for anemia, clotting issues, infection risk)
* EKG (especially if you're over 50 or have cardiac history)
* Chest X-ray (to rule out any lung issues)
* Urinalysis
* Possibly a COVID test or MRSA screening

If you have a heart condition or are on certain meds (like blood thinners), you might also need clearance from your cardiologist.

4. Meet the Anesthesiologist (or Their Rep)

This is when you talk about how they'll knock you out—or not:

* General anesthesia: You're fully unconscious
* Regional anesthesia: Nerve blocks, spinal or epidural (you're awake but numbed)
* Sedation + Local: For smaller procedures

They'll ask:

* Have you ever had trouble waking up from anesthesia?
* Any history of nausea or vomiting after surgery?
* Do you use alcohol, nicotine, or recreational drugs? (Be honest—it affects anesthesia.)

"It was the anesthesiologist who caught that I had sleep apnea," said James, 71, *"and they adjusted the meds. I might've avoided complications because of that conversation."*

Questions They'll Ask You (and You Should Ask Them)

They'll want to know:

* "Who will drive you home?"
* "Do you live alone?"
* "Do you have stairs in your home?"
* "Will someone stay with you after surgery?"
* "Do you use assistive devices—canes, walkers?"

Packing Tips, Mental Prep, and All the Weird Stuff Nobody Told You About

You should ask:

* "How long will I be under anesthesia?"
* "Will I get antibiotics before or after surgery?"
* "What kind of pain meds will I get?"
* "Do I need to stop taking any of my medications before surgery?"

Medication Madness: What to Pause, What to Keep

One of the biggest—and most important—parts of the pre-op appointment is reviewing which medications and supplements you need to pause before surgery. Why? Because some drugs increase your risk of bleeding, affect how anesthesia works, or mess with your vital signs.

Medications you may need to stop:

- Blood thinners (e.g., aspirin, warfarin, Plavix)
- Certain anti-inflammatory drugs (NSAIDs like ibuprofen or naproxen
- Herbal supplements (especially ginkgo, ginseng, garlic, turmeric, St. John's Wort)
- Some diabetes medications

Your surgical team will give you a tailored "stop/start" list—read it carefully and ask questions if anything's unclear.

Logistics, Baby

This is the time to sort out:

* Surgery time and location
* Arrival time and fasting instructions
* What to bring and wear
* Discharge plans (Are you going home the same day? Staying overnight?)

Also, you may be given:

* Pre-op bathing kits with antimicrobial soap

* Nutrition advice, like high-protein shakes to drink in the days before surgery
* Consent forms to sign—read them!

How You Might Feel (Emotionally)

There's no getting around this: the pre-op appointment makes things real. That surgery that was months away is now a blinking light on your calendar.

People describe feeling:

* Excited to finally fix the problem
* Nervous about complications
* Overwhelmed by information
* Tense over time off work, family care, or financial logistics

Some cry in the car afterward. Some go home and rearrange their kitchen. Others, like Carla, binge-watch "Grey's Anatomy" and regret it immediately.

This is all normal.

Your Assignment: Be a Partner in Your Prep

This isn't just the medical team's job. You have a role, too. Here's what to do after the appointment:

- Follow the medication instructions to the letter
- Get any extra tests or consults done ASAP
- Arrange your support system (drivers, caregivers, pet sitters)
- Set up your home for easy mobility (more on that in Chapter 5!)
- And if anything feels off—call your team right away.

As Carla told me, weeks after her knee replacement:

"That pre-op appointment felt overwhelming at the time. But afterward? I felt seen. I felt ready. Like this wasn't happening to me—I was part of it."

And you are. You're not just a patient—you're a partner in your healing.

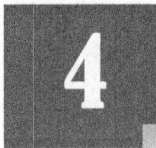

4 PREHABILITATION

Or, "Get Strong Now So You're Not Cussing Later"

The "Prehab" Secret Surgeons Don't Always Emphasize

When Tom, 59, was told he needed a knee replacement, his surgeon handed him a packet and said, "We'll see you in six weeks." No one mentioned exercise. No one said a word about strengthening. So Tom did what most people do—he waited.

Big mistake.

"Coming out of surgery, I felt like my leg had already given up on me," he told me. *"It was like waking up in a marathon I hadn't trained for."*

Contrast that with Dena, a 66-year-old retired teacher who spent four weeks doing targeted exercises with a physical therapist before her hip surgery.

"I was up with the walker the same day. I wasn't in pain-free bliss or anything, but I had power. I could feel it."

That power? That resilience? That's prehabilitation, or prehab—a fancy word for preparing your body for surgery so you can recover faster and better.

And if your surgeon hasn't brought it up yet, don't worry. We will.

What Is Prehab—and Why Does It Matter?

Packing Tips, Mental Prep, and All the Weird Stuff Nobody Told You About

Prehab is a proactive, short-term program of exercise, movement, and education designed to:

- Strengthen the muscles surrounding your surgical joint
- Improve balance and mobility
- Reduce pain
- Boost endurance and cardiovascular fitness
- Teach you how to move safely after surgery (getting up, using stairs, etc.)

It's the "training montage" part of your story. It may not be sexy, but it works. Multiple studies have shown that people who undergo prehab before joint surgery:

- Have faster recovery times
- Experience less post-op pain
- Need less rehab afterward
- Are less likely to need inpatient rehab (meaning they go home, not to a facility)

One study found that prehab reduced the need for post-surgical inpatient rehab by nearly 30% for total knee replacements. That's not just mobility—that's money, time, and emotional stress saved.

Why Surgeons Might Not Push It

This always surprises patients: your orthopedic surgeon might not emphasize prehab unless you ask. Why?

- Time constraints in appointments
- Assumptions that primary care or PT will handle it
- Focus on the surgery itself, not the lead-up
- Or sometimes, they're just not used to patients being this proactive

But the best surgeons are increasingly recommending it—especially for knees, hips, and shoulders, where support muscle is critical to recovery.

What Does Prehab Actually Look Like?

Jason M. Aucoin

It's usually a 2–6 week plan tailored to your joint, your abilities, and your surgery timeline. You can do it with a physical therapist, at a gym, or even at home—though having a PT guide the first few sessions is ideal.

Let's break it down by goals:

1. Build Strength Around the Joint

Your muscles will be called in as backup dancers once the joint is cut, stitched, or replaced. Prehab focuses on:

- Quads, glutes, hamstrings for knee/hip surgeries
- Deltoids, rotator cuff, scapular stabilizers for shoulder surgeries
- Core muscles for every kind of joint stability

Common moves:

- Seated leg extensions
- Straight-leg raises
- Mini squats or sit-to-stand drills
- Resistance band work
- Bridges (yes, you'll curse the bridges)

2. Improve Range of Motion

Going into surgery with stiff, tight muscles makes post-op mobility harder. Prehab includes:

- Gentle stretching
- Passive range of motion exercises
- Joint mobility drills (especially for shoulders and knees)

3. Build Cardiovascular Stamina

Surgery takes a toll. Walking, climbing stairs, and doing PT afterward takes energy.

Low-impact options like recumbent biking, elliptical, or swimming

Walking for increasing distances (even around the house)

Packing Tips, Mental Prep, and All the Weird Stuff Nobody Told You About

Breathing exercises and posture work

4. Practice Safe Movement Techniques

Especially important for joint replacements or for patients who live alone:

* How to use a walker or cane properly
* Getting out of bed, cars, and chairs without straining
* Navigating stairs or curbs
* Protecting the surgical site during daily movement

Dena's pro tip:

"My PT had me pretend to go to the bathroom one-legged using a walker. I was like, really? But after surgery? It saved me. I didn't panic."

5. Reduce Pain and Swelling

Some PTs will start gentle manual therapy (like massage or lymphatic drainage), or ice/heat regimens to reduce inflammation before the procedure. The idea is to:

* Calm the area down
* Get blood flowing
* Improve tissue quality

Do You Need a Physical Therapist?

Ideally, yes. At least for one or two sessions. Here's why:

* They assess your baseline function
* They'll create a safe, effective program
* They teach movement mechanics (like how to protect your healing joint)
* They spot weaknesses or imbalances you can't see

If insurance is a concern, ask about group prehab classes (some hospitals offer them), or see if your surgeon's office has a recommended pre-op program.

Jason M. Aucoin

What If You Can't Exercise Much?

Not everyone can—or should—dive into a gym routine. If you're in severe pain, have mobility limits, or other health issues, prehab can be adapted:

- Chair-based strength work
- Gentle resistance bands
- Breathing and isometric exercises
- Nutrition and mindset coaching (yes, that counts)

Even small efforts matter. Prehab isn't about becoming a bodybuilder—it's about making surgery less of a knockout punch.

Real Talk: It Might Hurt... a Little

Prehab isn't always comfortable. You're moving a joint that already hurts. But unlike "pushing through pain" post-surgery (which can be risky), this discomfort is usually safe—and even helpful.

You should never feel sharp, stabbing, or severe pain. But mild soreness the next day? Totally normal.

As Tom (the guy who skipped prehab) told me when he finally tried it before his second knee surgery:

"It sucked, honestly. But my recovery after the second knee was like night and day. I'd do it again in a heartbeat."

Other Elements of Prehab You Shouldn't Ignore

* Nutrition: Load up on protein and anti-inflammatory foods now
* Sleep: Start improving sleep quality (you'll need that energy banked)
* Mental prep: Meditation, mindfulness, or therapy—surgery is physical and emotional
* Logistics: Use this time to prep your home for recovery (we cover that in Chapter 5!)

Bottom Line: Train Like You're Coming Back Stronger

Packing Tips, Mental Prep, and All the Weird Stuff Nobody Told You About

Surgery may be the main event, but prehab is the training camp. It's your chance to take some control in a process that often feels like a medical conveyor belt.

It doesn't need to be complicated or intense. It just needs to be intentional.

Dena's advice to anyone heading into joint surgery?

"Don't wait for the pain to go away. Build the strength that'll carry you through it."

And that's what prehab is really about—carrying yourself through the hard part and into healing.

5

MEDS, DIET, & HOME PREP

Or, "Don't Trip Over Your Dog with a Knee Brace On"

The Not-So-Secret Ingredient of a Smooth Recovery

Let's be honest—when people talk about preparing for joint surgery, they usually picture squats, paperwork, or maybe rearranging their Netflix queue for the couch-bound days ahead.

But the truth? One of the most underrated superpowers in your surgery prep toolkit is your environment.

And your meds.

And your food.

In other words: your internal and external setup can determine whether recovery is a slog or a smoother ride.

And the best part? These are things you can control.

Medications — Your Pre-Surgical Chemistry Check

The "Don't-Take List" (Seriously, Don't)

Certain medications, vitamins, and supplements can increase your risk of bleeding, mess with anesthesia, or interfere with healing. Your surgical team will give you specific guidance, but here's the general rule of thumb:

Packing Tips, Mental Prep, and All the Weird Stuff Nobody Told You About

Start adjusting about 7–10 days before surgery.

Here's what's often paused:

- Blood thinners: aspirin, warfarin (Coumadin), clopidogrel (Plavix)
- NSAIDs: ibuprofen (Advil), naproxen (Aleve), diclofenac
- Herbal supplements: ginkgo, garlic, ginseng, turmeric, St. John's Wort
- Fish oil, vitamin E (in large doses)

Pro Tip:

Write down everything you take—prescriptions, over-the-counter meds, gummies, powders, essential oils, moon water. Whatever. Your doctor needs the full picture.

The "Keep-Taking List" (With a Few Caveats)

Some medications should not be stopped. This usually includes:

- Blood pressure meds
- Thyroid meds
- Some heart medications
- Certain diabetes meds (though dosing may be adjusted)

Your anesthesia team may give you exact timing—for example, taking meds with a sip of water a few hours before surgery.

"I almost skipped my blood pressure pill the morning of," said Wayne, 67, "because I thought I wasn't supposed to eat or drink anything. Luckily, my nurse caught it. Could've been a problem."

Ask specifically:

- "Which meds do I keep taking right up to surgery?"
- "Which ones do I stop—and when?"
- "Can I take supplements again after surgery? When?"

Your Pre-Op Diet — Fuel the Healing Machine

Can't Bend? Can't Snap? Can't Stop Laughing!

Jason M. Aucoin

No, you don't need to go keto or juice for seven days. But what you eat in the weeks before surgery can make a real difference in your inflammation levels, immune system, and energy stores for healing.

The Goals Are Simple:

- Boost your immune system
- Reduce inflammation
- Support tissue repair
- Prevent constipation (hello, pain meds)
- Maintain strength and stamina

```
Foods to Prioritize:
```

- Lean proteins: chicken, fish, eggs, tofu, Greek yogurt
- Colorful vegetables: spinach, broccoli, bell peppers, sweet potatoes
- Anti-inflammatory fats: olive oil, avocado, walnuts, flaxseed
- Whole grains: oats, brown rice, quinoa
- Hydration: water, herbal teas, broths

If your doctor gave you a protein shake or nutritional supplement to drink in the days before surgery, use it. Research has shown these pre-op nutrition shakes can lower infection risks and improve outcomes.

"I drank this vanilla shake for three days before my surgery," said Carla, 63. *"Wasn't gourmet, but I'd drink dog food if it meant fewer complications."*

```
Foods to Limit or Avoid:
```

- Highly processed snacks
- Sugary drinks
- Excess salt (can cause bloating and fluid retention)
- Alcohol (interferes with medications and healing)
- Red meat and fried foods (harder to digest, pro-inflammatory)

A Word on Constipation

Yes, we're going there. Pain meds—especially opioids—slow everything down.

Packing Tips, Mental Prep, and All the Weird Stuff Nobody Told You About

Start now by:

- Increasing fiber (fruits, veggies, chia seeds)
- Drinking water
- Considering a mild stool softener (with your doc's okay)

You'll thank yourself when you're not clutching the bathroom wall post-op.

Home Prep — Design Your Recovery Nest

Your home isn't just where you live—it's where you'll heal. So making it recovery-friendly is one of the smartest, kindest things you can do for future you.

Here's how to get started:

1. Declutter Like a Safety Inspector

- Clear walkways of cords, rugs, shoes, and dog toys (aka ankle mines)
- Secure slippery rugs or remove them altogether
- Make space around the bed, couch, and bathroom

If you're having lower body surgery, stairs will be your arch nemesis. Try to set up a main floor recovery zone with:

* Bed or recliner
* Access to a bathroom
* Meds, snacks, and phone charger within arm's reach

2. Stock Up On Essentials

You don't want to send your partner or kid out for stool softener at midnight. Get these ahead of time:

- Prescriptions (pain meds, antibiotics, stool softeners, anti nausea)
- Ice packs or cold therapy machines
- Compression socks (if recommended)

Can't Bend? Can't Snap? Can't Stop Laughing!

- Easy-to-prep meals (frozen burritos are underrated
- Non-slip socks or slipper
- Reachers, long-handled shoehorns, raised toilet seats (you'll get the full list later in the book)

"My biggest win?" said Marisol, 70. "A bedside commode. Glamorous? No. But I didn't have to climb stairs in the middle of the night."

3. Prep Your Wardrobe

Skip the skinny jeans and tight tees. You'll want:

- Loose, breathable clothing
- Easy pull-on pants or shorts
- Zip-up or button-up tops (especially for shoulder/elbow surgeries)
- Slippers or shoes with a back and good grip

4. Plan Your Support Team

Even if you live alone, you shouldn't recover alone. Think through:

- Who can drive you home after surgery?
- Who can stay with you for the first 24–72 hours?
- Who can check on you, bring groceries, or help with pets?
- If your friends or family say, "Let me know if you need anything," hand them a list.

5. The Emotional Side of Prep

This part often gets ignored—but prepping your mind is just as important.

- Journal your fears and questions
- Watch surgery prep videos from reputable sources (some hospitals have these)
- Talk to someone who's had the surgery
- Don't hesitate to ask your doctor the "what ifs" that are keeping you up at night

"I spent more time worrying than preparing," said James, 72. "Next time, I'd schedule time to do both."

Packing Tips, Mental Prep, and All the Weird Stuff Nobody Told You About

The Final Days Before Surgery: Check, Check, Double-Check

Here's your 3-day countdown list:

- Pick up all prescriptions
- Stop or adjust meds as directed
- Fill the fridge and freezer
- Do laundry (you'll want clean, comfy clothes)
- Set up your recovery zone
- Line up rides and help
- Do a trial run with your walker or crutches
- Take pre-op nutrition drinks if recommended
- Ask final questions at your pre-op appointment

You've Got This—And You're Not Alone

Preparing for joint surgery isn't just about what happens in the OR. It's about what happens at home, in your body, and in your mind. And while it might feel like a lot now, every effort you make in advance pays dividends in your recovery.

You're not over preparing—you're building your comeback.

"I felt proud of my setup," said Dena. "It was like I made a little recovery castle. I wasn't just lying around—I was healing on purpose."

And so are you.

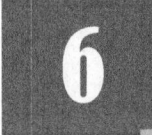

THE NIGHT BEFORE

Or, "Trying to Sleep While Mentally Replaying Every Worst-Case Scenario"

Let's Talk About the Night Before

You've checked off the lists. You've rearranged furniture, paused meds, packed your surgery bag. You've done your prehab (hopefully) and stocked up on frozen meals, podcasts, and those weird bendy straws.

But then the clock ticks closer to surgery morning.

And suddenly, your brain won't shut up.

Even the most prepared people—those who've faced childbirth, broken bones, and marathon finals—will tell you: the night before surgery is its own psychological rodeo.

What This Chapter Is Really About

Yes, we'll go over final steps—what to do, what not to eat, what to pack. But this chapter isn't just about checking boxes. It's about naming what happens to us emotionally when the house is quiet, and you're lying there, staring at the ceiling, wondering:

> *What if something goes wrong? What if I come out worse than I went in?*

We're going to hold space for that. And we're going to walk through it.

Packing Tips, Mental Prep, and All the Weird Stuff Nobody Told You About

Because you're not alone in feeling this way.

What to Do the Night Before Surgery

`1. Follow Your Pre-Surgery Eating & Drinking Instructions`

Most hospitals follow the "nothing by mouth after midnight" rule—but it varies:
- Some allow clear liquids up to 2–4 hours before surgery
- Some want you to avoid even water
- Some give you a pre-op carb drink (yep, that's a thing)

Ask your surgical team for exact instructions. And follow them. Eating or drinking too late could mean your surgery gets postponed.

"I forgot and took a sip of coffee at 6 a.m.," said Nora, 58. "They had to bump me to the next day. I cried in the parking lot."

`2. Shower As Directed (Yes, With the Weird Soap)`

You'll likely be asked to shower with an antibacterial soap the night before and possibly the morning of surgery. The most common: chlorhexidine gluconate (Hibiclens).

- Don't use it on your face, genitals, or open wounds
- Let it sit on your skin for about a minute before rinsing
- Avoid lotions, powders, or deodorants after

Why the fuss? Reducing skin bacteria helps prevent infection after surgery.

Is it drying and mildly unpleasant? Yep. But it works.

`3. Pack Your Surgery Bag (Even for Outpatient Procedures)`

Jason M. Aucoin

You don't need a steamer trunk. But you do want to feel comfortable, in control, and not reliant on hospital socks for dignity.

Here's a solid go-bag list:

- Photo ID and insurance card
- Any paperwork you've been asked to bring
- List of your meds and allergies
- Phone + charger
- Glasses/hearing aids/dentures if needed
- A book, journal, or calming distraction
- Comfy clothes for post-op (loose, soft, easy on/off)
- Slip-on shoes
- Lip balm and lotion (hospitals = dry city)

If you're staying overnight:
- CPAP if you use one
- A few familiar comforts: small pillow, cozy socks, your own blanket (if allowed)

4. Set Up Morning Logistics
- Confirm your ride
- Set alarms (more than one!)
- Lay out clothes
- Review instructions one last time
- Try not to freak out (more on that below)

Now, Let's Talk About the Mental Stuff

Because this is the part no one preps you for. You can have your Hibiclens, your soft pants, and your emergency jello cups—and still find yourself wide awake, spiraling.

That's normal. Let's unpack it.

The Emotional Cocktail of the Night Before Surgery

1. Fear (Totally Rational, By the Way)
Fear of:

- Pain
- Complications
- Anesthesia
- Not waking up
- Waking up mid-surgery (spoiler: it's extremely rare)
- Loss of independence
- Not bouncing back like you hope

Even if the stats are in your favor (they usually are), you're allowed to be scared. You're putting your body in someone else's hands. That's a big deal.

2. Grief
Many people don't realize what they're feeling is grief:
- Grieving your old body
- Your pre-surgery independence
- The loss of mobility or function
- Even just the sadness of needing surgery in the first place

That's okay. You're not "too emotional." You're a human having a human reaction to something big.

3. Hope (But It's the Quiet Kind)
There's hope in there too, though it might whisper. Hope that:
- This will relieve your pain
- You'll move freely again
- You'll get your life back

Sometimes it hides behind fear and frustration, but it's there. Keep feeding it.

What Can You Do With All That Emotion?

Here are some tools that help real patients (and maybe you too):

1. Journal—Even Just a Few Lines
Write down:
- What you're feeling

Can't Bend? Can't Snap? Can't Stop Laughing!

Jason M. Aucoin
- What you're afraid of
- What you're hoping for
- Who or what you're grateful for

"I wrote a letter to my body," said Alan, 64. "Thanking it for getting me this far. Cheesy, maybe, but it grounded me."

2. Breathe With Purpose
Inhale 4 counts. Hold 4. Exhale 6. Repeat. It activates your parasympathetic nervous system—the calm-down response.

Even five minutes helps. Add calming music if you want.

3. Do Something Normal
Watch a comfort show. Brush your teeth to your favorite song. Snuggle your dog. These tiny routines are proof: life still goes on. You're still you.

4. Talk to Someone Who Gets It
Call a friend who's had surgery. Ask them how they felt the night before. Most will say the same thing:

"It was harder in my head than it was in reality."

And that's true for a lot of people. The anticipation is often worse than the actual surgery and recovery.

If You Can't Sleep... That's Normal Too

Don't beat yourself up for being awake at 2 a.m. Your body is in alert mode. That's a survival feature.

What can help:
- Gentle meditation apps
- Progressive muscle relaxation (tense and release each muscle group)
- Audiobooks or nature sounds
- Scented oils like lavender or eucalyptus

Packing Tips, Mental Prep, and All the Weird Stuff Nobody Told You About

And if you're still awake at 4 a.m.? You'll still get through surgery just fine. The anesthesiologist's got your back. Sleep deprivation doesn't cancel recovery—it just makes you slightly more likely to nap hard afterward.

The Morning Will Come

You're here. You've prepared, packed, cleaned, journaled, cried, maybe panicked a little—and you're still here.

Surgery is hard. But you're not going into this powerless.

You've equipped yourself with knowledge. You've created a healing space. You've asked the hard questions. You've done the work.

So let the morning come.

Let the body rest, even if it's not sleeping.

Let hope speak a little louder than fear.

And when you wake up in the recovery room, groggy and sore but on the other side, you'll have earned every inch of the peace that follows.

Jason M. Aucoin

PART TWO
SURGERY BY JOINT

Packing Tips, Mental Prep, and All the Weird Stuff Nobody Told You About

7

KNEE SURGERY – PRE & POST BREAKDOWN

Or, "So Your Knee Quit Its Job—Let's Help It Clock Back In"

Anatomy of the Knee Joint

Before We Cut, Let's Understand What's Inside

Imagine your knee as the body's busiest intersection—carrying weight, absorbing shock, bending, straightening, twisting, stopping, and starting. Unlike a simple hinge, the knee is more like a live-action construction site of bones, ligaments, cartilage, and fluid, all working to keep you upright and moving.

Here's the crew:

- Bones: The knee joint is formed where three bones meet:
  - Femur (thighbone)
  - Tibia (shinbone)
  - Patella (kneecap)

- Cartilage:
  - Articular cartilage covers bone surfaces, reducing friction.
  - Menisci (medial and lateral) are C-shaped shock absorbers between femur and tibia.

- Ligaments:

Can't Bend? Can't Snap? Can't Stop Laughing!

- ACL (anterior cruciate ligament) and PCL (posterior) stabilize front-to-back movement.
- MCL (medial) and LCL (lateral) control side-to-side motion.

- Tendons: Connect muscle to bone, especially the quadriceps tendon and patellar tendon.

- Synovial Fluid: Think WD-40 for your knee. It keeps everything slick and functional.

This complexity makes the knee strong—but also vulnerable. And when one part breaks down, it affects the whole system.

Common Knee Conditions Requiring Surgery

When Ice, Physical Therapy, and Bracing Just Don't Cut It Anymore

Knee surgery isn't a first resort—it's usually the last card after conservative treatments have failed. But when pain persists, mobility suffers, or instability interferes with daily life, surgery becomes a powerful option for healing and function.

Let's break down the three major categories of knee surgeries and what they're all about.

ACL/PCL Tears and Reconstruction

The Story of Snaps, Pivots, and Sudden "Pops"

The ACL and PCL are two ligaments deep inside the knee. They crisscross like a pair of ropes, preventing your tibia from sliding too far forward or backward.

- Who tears these?
- Athletes (especially soccer, football, basketball, skiing)
- Weekend warriors in pick-up games
- Anyone who's twisted wrong on stairs or uneven ground

"I felt a pop and dropped," said Ryan, 28. *"I thought someone kicked me, but no one was there."*

Packing Tips, Mental Prep, and All the Weird Stuff Nobody Told You About

- Surgery Overview:
- Involves reconstructing (not repairing) the ligament using a graft—either from your own body (hamstring, patellar tendon) or a donor.
- Often done arthroscopically (small incisions + camera).
- Recovery takes 6 to 12 months, depending on the sport or activity you want to return to.

Pre-op tip:
- "Prehab" is crucial. The stronger your quads and hamstrings, the smoother the post-op recovery.

- Post-op reality:
- Crutches and brace for a few weeks
- Aggressive physical therapy to restore range and strength
- Mental game: trusting the knee again takes longer than you'd think

Meniscus Injuries and Repair

Torn Cartilage Doesn't Have to Mean Torn Dreams

The meniscus is like the knee's shock absorber. Each knee has two, and they're essential for cushioning and stability. But they're also prone to tears—either suddenly (sports injury) or gradually (degeneration over time).

- Symptoms of a tear:
- Sharp pain with twisting
- Swelling within 24–48 hours
- Clicking or catching
- Difficulty squatting or going downstairs

- Surgery Types:
- Meniscectomy (partial removal of the torn portion): quicker recovery, but less cartilage means more wear later.
- Meniscus repair (suturing the tear): preferred in younger patients, but longer healing.

"I was hiking in the Rockies six months after my repair," said Denise, 43. "Slow and steady, but pain-free."

- Recovery timelines:
- Meniscectomy: 2–6 weeks

Can't Bend? Can't Snap? Can't Stop Laughing!

- Repair: 3–6 months, sometimes longer depending on tear location and blood supply

Patellar Issues and Solutions

When Your Kneecap Doesn't Want to Stay in Its Lane

The patella (kneecap) glides in a groove at the front of the femur. But sometimes it gets off-track, causing pain, instability, or even dislocation.

- Common conditions:
- Patellofemoral pain syndrome: overuse or misalignment
- Patellar instability: recurrent dislocations
- Cartilage damage behind the kneecap

- Surgical Options May Include:
- Lateral release: cutting tight tissue pulling the patella sideways
- Realignment procedures: shifting the tendon or bone to stabilize movement
- Chondroplasty or cartilage grafts for smoothing damaged surfaces

"My knee kept sliding out of place," said Kelly, 33. "After the realignment surgery, I could finally trust it again."

- Recovery Considerations:
- Weight-bearing and range of motion restrictions
- Quad strengthening is key to keeping the patella where it belongs
- Bracing and taping may be used during recovery

Every Knee Surgery Is a Partnership

Surgeons can do remarkable things with scalpels, scopes, and sutures—but what you do before and after surgery is just as critical.

- Prehab builds the foundation
- Surgery fixes the structure
- Rehab restores the function
- You bring the effort, patience, and mindset

Preoperative Preparation and Planning

Or, "How to Become Your Own Best Surgical Assistant"

Think of knee surgery as a tag-team relay race. Your surgeon carries the baton for the operation itself—but you're responsible for the lap before and after. And trust us: a well-prepared patient often recovers faster, with fewer complications.

So how do you get prepped like a pro?
Packing Tips, Mental Prep, and All the Weird Stuff Nobody Told You About

1. Get to Know Your Knee (and Your Plan)
Ask your surgeon:
- What exactly are you fixing?
- What type of surgery will you do—and why?
- What are the risks and benefits?
- How long will I be on crutches?
- Can I drive afterwards? When?

Pro Tip: Take notes or bring someone to do it for you. Most patients remember only about 50% of what's said at pre-op consults. Nerves mess with memory.

2. Prehabilitation (Yes, Again!)

We touched on it in Chapter 4, but let's hammer it home:

"The stronger you go into surgery, the stronger you come out."

Prehab includes:
- Quad and hamstring strengthening
- Range-of-motion work
- Gentle cardio (stationary bike, swimming, etc.)

Many surgeons now require prehab because it improves outcomes—and because weak, tight muscles are like trying to build a house on a swamp.

3. Blood Work, Imaging, and Clearance
Expect:
- Labs (CBC, electrolytes, clotting factors)
- EKG (especially over age 50 or with a cardiac history)
- Chest X-ray (sometimes)
- Medical clearance from your primary doctor

They're checking that you're a safe candidate for anesthesia and surgery. It's not busywork—it's baseline safety.

4. Home Prep: Your Recovery HQ
Think about:
- Removing trip hazards (rugs, cords, loose pets)
- Setting up a sleeping space on the ground floor
- Installing grab bars, raised toilet seats, or a shower chair
- Stocking up on ice packs or a cold therapy machine
- Arranging help for the first 72 hours

Can't Bend? Can't Snap? Can't Stop Laughing!

Also, get your pharmacy involved early. Fill prescriptions before surgery so you're not scrambling while doped up on pain meds.

Surgical Approaches and Techniques

Arthroscopic Procedures

Small Tools, Big Results

Arthroscopy is minimally invasive surgery using a tiny camera (arthroscope) and slender instruments inserted through small incisions. Think of it as keyhole surgery for the knee.

Common Arthroscopic Procedures:
- Meniscus repair or removal
- ACL reconstruction
- Cartilage debridement
- Removal of loose bodies or inflamed tissue

Pros:
- Smaller incisions
- Less post-op pain
- Faster recovery
- Lower infection risk

"I walked with a cane the next day," said Marcus, 47, after his arthroscopic meniscectomy. *"Still sore, but amazed."*

Cons:
- Not suitable for every condition (complex tears or deformities may need open surgery)
- Still requires anesthesia and rehab—don't let the size of the incisions fool you

Open Knee Surgery

The Bigger Cut with Bigger Goals

Open knee surgery involves a larger incision to access the joint. It's more invasive but sometimes necessary—especially for complex reconstructions or total knee replacements.

When It's Used:
- Total or partial knee replacement
- Severe patellar instability procedures
- Multi-ligament reconstructions

- Tumor removal or fracture repairs

Pros:
- Better visibility for the surgeon
- Ideal for complex or multi-structure repairs

Cons:
- More tissue trauma
- Longer healing time
- Higher risk of blood clots or infection

"My total knee replacement was no joke," said Caroline, 62. "But four months later, I danced at my granddaughter's wedding. Worth every painful step."

Immediate Post-Operative Care

The First 48 Hours: Ice, Elevate, Repeat

Post-op care is about two things: managing pain and preventing complications. Whether you had arthroscopy or open surgery, the first 2–3 days are critical.

1. Pain Management
You'll likely get a combo of:
- Oral opioids (short term)
- NSAIDs (to reduce inflammation)
- Ice or cold therapy
- Elevation (above heart level)
- Compression wrap or knee brace

Nerve blocks or spinal anesthesia may reduce immediate post-op pain significantly—but it'll wear off, and you'll need a backup plan.

"When the block wore off at 2 a.m., I thought I'd been hit by a bus," said Juan, 55. "Take your meds before the pain catches up."

2. Wound Care
- Keep the bandage dry and intact
- Don't soak the incision (no baths or swimming)
- Watch for redness, pus, or foul odor
- Notify your surgeon for fevers or excessive swelling

3. Movement (Yes, Already)

Can't Bend? Can't Snap? Can't Stop Laughing!

Jason M. Aucoin

Many patients are up and walking with assistance the same day or next morning. Early mobility helps prevent:
- Blood clots
- Pneumonia
- Joint stiffness

You'll likely be started on ankle pumps, heel slides, or even assisted standing with a walker or crutches before you leave the hospital.

Rehabilitation Timeline and Protocols

The Real Work Starts Here

Recovery is a team sport—and you're the captain.

Rehab timelines vary by procedure, but here's a general idea:

Week 1-2: Healing and Basic Motion
- Ice, elevate, rest
- Gentle range-of-motion exercises
- Begin physical therapy (supervised or at home)
- Weight-bearing as directed (from toe-touch to full, depending on procedure)

"My therapist made me bend my knee on Day 3. I cried—but it worked," said Ella, 68.

Week 3-6: Gaining Strength and Stability
- Increase range of motion (goal: 90° flexion or more)
- Strengthen quads, hamstrings, glutes
- Gait training
- Stationary bike or pool therapy

Weeks 7-12: Real-Life Movement
- Advance to bodyweight exercises
- Balance work
- Light stair climbing
- Treadmill walking or elliptical
- Start weaning off brace/crutches

Month 3-6+: Return to Function (and Life)
- Sport-specific drills (if cleared)
- Full range of motion expected
- Return to hiking, driving, or higher-impact tasks
- Ongoing strengthening for injury prevention

Packing Tips, Mental Prep, and All the Weird Stuff Nobody Told You About

"I'm not just walking—I'm back to playing tennis," said Julie, 59, six months post-ACL reconstruction. *"Rehab was brutal, but so worth it."*

Can't Bend? Can't Snap? Can't Stop Laughing!

8. Hip Surgery — Prep & Recovery Tips

Or, "Getting Hip to Hip Surgery"

Hip Joint Anatomy and Biomechanics

Why Your Hip Is Basically a Deep-Sea Submarine Hatch—Only Cooler

The hip is one of the most elegant and powerful joints in the body. Think of it as a highly engineered ball-and-socket design, meant to handle a lifetime of force, rotation, and weight-bearing—while allowing you to sprint, squat, dance, and sit cross-legged at yoga (or at least try).

Key Structures:

- Femoral Head: The ball at the top of the thighbone (femur).
- Acetabulum: The socket in the pelvis that houses the femoral head.
- Labrum: A ring of cartilage that deepens the socket and adds stability.
- Articular Cartilage: Covers the surfaces of the ball and socket, reducing friction.
- Ligaments and Capsule: Tough bands that keep the joint secure.
- Muscles: The glutes, hip flexors, adductors, and external rotators all work together like a symphony to move and stabilize.

The biomechanics of the hip allow three planes of motion—flexion/extension, abduction/adduction, and rotation—making it incredibly versatile but also vulnerable to breakdown.

Common Hip Pathologies

Packing Tips, Mental Prep, and All the Weird Stuff Nobody Told You About

When Your Hip Becomes a Real Pain in the... You Know

Osteoarthritis of the Hip

"Bone on Bone" and What That Really Means

Osteoarthritis (OA) is the wear-and-tear version of joint breakdown. Over time, the smooth cartilage wears away, the joint space narrows, and the bones start rubbing—causing stiffness, pain, and a crunchy grinding sound (called crepitus).

Who Gets It?
- People over 50
- Athletes with previous injuries
- Folks with family history or abnormal hip shapes

Symptoms:
- Groin pain (not outer hip—surprise!)
- Stiffness after sitting
- Trouble tying shoes or getting in/out of cars
- Limping or reduced walking distance

Treatment Often Leads To: Total Hip Replacement (THR) – a life-changing surgery that swaps the damaged joint with a prosthetic one.

"Before my hip replacement, I couldn't stand for more than 10 minutes," said Greg, 64. *"Afterward? I walked two miles by week six."*

Hip Labral Tears

When the Hip's Cartilage Ring Fails to Keep the Party Going

The labrum is the cartilage rim that seals the ball inside the socket. When it tears—often due to trauma, overuse, or anatomical quirks—it can cause pain, clicking, and instability.

Common in:
- Dancers, gymnasts, and hockey players
- People with FAI (see below)
- Those with previous hip injuries

Symptoms:
- Sharp groin or lateral hip pain
- Clicking or locking sensation

Can't Bend? Can't Snap? Can't Stop Laughing!

Jason M. Aucoin
- Pain when sitting or rotating the hip
- Limited range of motion

Surgical Solution:
Hip Arthroscopy — the labrum can be repaired or debrided using small incisions and a camera.

Femoroacetabular Impingement (FAI)

AKA: The Bones Are Fighting Each Other

FAI occurs when the femoral head and/or acetabulum have abnormal shapes that cause them to pinch during movement—often damaging the labrum in the process.

Types of FAI:
- Cam: extra bone on femoral head
- Pincer: overcoverage of socket
- Combined: a frustrating combo platter

Symptoms:
- Groin pain with activity
- Stiffness and limited motion
- Pain after prolonged sitting
- Clicking or catching

Surgical Treatment:
FAI can often be corrected via arthroscopy, where excess bone is shaved and the labrum repaired.

"I had a Cam impingement and didn't even know it," said Jenna, 35. "Fixing it gave me my yoga practice back."

Preoperative Assessment and Planning

Staging the Show Before the Scalpel Enters

Just like with knee surgery, proper preparation is half the battle. But hip surgery often requires more detailed planning because of the joint's deep location and involvement in nearly every movement we make.

1. Imaging and Diagnosis
Expect to undergo:
- X-rays: to assess joint space and bony deformities
- MRI or MR arthrogram: for soft tissue issues like labral tears
- CT scans: in complex cases, to build a surgical map

Packing Tips, Mental Prep, and All the Weird Stuff Nobody Told You About

"My CT showed the exact spot of the impingement," said Theo, 29. *"It was like a blueprint for my surgeon."*

2. Surgical Decision-Making

Questions your surgeon will cover:
- Is arthroscopy appropriate, or is a full replacement needed?
- What implants or prosthetics will be used?
- Are there pre-existing conditions (like scoliosis or leg length differences) that complicate the plan?

3. Prehabilitation

Yes, again! For hips, it focuses on:
- Gluteal and core strengthening
- Flexibility (hip flexors, hamstrings, piriformis)
- Gait training
- Reducing compensation patterns

Why it matters: Stronger muscles and better movement patterns pre-op mean better protection for your new hip or repaired joint post-op.

4. Lifestyle Prep

- Arrange for someone to help for the first 5–7 days.
- Stock up on high-protein meals and hydration aids.
- Make your recovery zone accessible—avoid stairs at first.
- Prepare loose clothing (you won't want skinny jeans after hip surgery, trust us).
- Plan for at least 4–6 weeks off work for major procedures.

"I underestimated how much help I'd need in the first week," said Lauren, 51. *"Swallowing my pride and asking for help made all the difference."*

Surgical Approaches

Or: "Three Roads to Your Hip, and Why Your Surgeon Picks One Over the Other"

When it comes to hip surgery, particularly total hip replacements, the approach your surgeon chooses matters—not just during the operation, but in your recovery, risk of dislocation, and even where your scar ends up.

So let's break it down, one incision at a time.

Can't Bend? Can't Snap? Can't Stop Laughing!

Jason M. Aucoin
Anterior Approach

Front and Center

This approach goes through the front of the hip, between natural muscle planes—meaning no muscles are cut, just retracted.

Pros:
- Muscle-sparing
- Typically less post-op pain
- Faster initial recovery
- Smaller incision, less limping early on
- Lower dislocation risk in some patients

Cons:
- Steep learning curve for surgeons
- Not suitable for every body type (obesity, abnormal anatomy)
- Risk of injury to lateral femoral cutaneous nerve (can cause thigh numbness)

Who It's Best For:
Active adults, people prioritizing a quicker early recovery, and anyone with good anatomy for anterior access.

"I was walking without a cane in two weeks," said Barry, 57, who had an anterior THR. "It felt like a fast-forward button on healing."

Posterior Approach

Old Faithful

The most traditional route—through the back of the hip. Some muscle is cut, particularly the short external rotators, to expose the joint.

Pros:
- Excellent visibility for the surgeon
- Works well in larger patients or complex anatomy
- Widely practiced—surgeons are very experienced with it

Cons:
- Muscle healing takes longer
- Slightly higher dislocation risk (especially during early recovery)
- Avoiding certain movements (like bending past 90°) post-op is essential

Who It's Best For:
Patients with complex hip issues, revision surgeries, or when other approaches aren't feasible.

Packing Tips, Mental Prep, and All the Weird Stuff Nobody Told You About

Lateral Approach

The Side Door

This route cuts through some of the hip abductors (like the gluteus medius) to access the joint.

Pros:
- Lower dislocation risk
- Good for balancing implant placement

Cons:
- Can cause temporary or persistent limp
- Muscle weakness is more common
- Less common in the U.S., so not all surgeons favor it

Who It's Best For:
Select cases where stability is critical, or in patients with high fall risk.

"My surgeon chose lateral because of my osteoporosis," said Helen, 70. "I had more rehab to do, but haven't had a single instability issue."

Hip Arthroscopy vs. Open Procedures

Small Tools vs. Full Access: When Minimally Invasive Isn't Enough

Hip Arthroscopy

This is the "scope" procedure—minimally invasive, using a camera and tools through small incisions.

Used For:
- Labral tears
- FAI
- Loose bodies
- Cartilage injuries
- Some early-stage arthritis

Recovery: Faster and less painful, but rehab is still critical. Weight-bearing may be restricted initially.

Open Hip Procedures
More invasive surgeries include:
- Total hip replacement (THR)

Can't Bend? Can't Snap? Can't Stop Laughing!

Jason M. Aucoin
- Hip resurfacing
- Periacetabular osteotomy (PAO)
- Complex reconstructions

Used For:
- Severe arthritis
- Bone deformities
- Advanced FAI or dysplasia
- Revision surgeries

Recovery: Longer due to muscle cutting and larger incisions. Hospital stays are usually 1–3 days.

"My arthroscopy was outpatient," said Dana, 33. "But after my total hip, I was in the hospital two nights and used a walker for a week."

Post-Operative Protocols by Procedure Type

From Ice Packs to Stair Climbs

Recovery isn't one-size-fits-all. Here's how it typically breaks down:

After Total Hip Replacement (THR):
- Day 1–2: Up and walking with assistance. Begin ankle pumps and isometric exercises.
- Week 1–2: Progress to cane/walker. Pain management, gentle PT.
- Week 3–6: Focus on hip strength, range of motion, gait correction.
- Week 6–12: Resume most daily activities. Return to work (desk jobs).
- 3–6 months: Resume low-impact sports (golf, swimming). Full strength returns gradually.

Restrictions: Depending on approach, you may have to avoid hip flexion past 90°, internal rotation, or crossing legs.

After Hip Arthroscopy:
- First Week: Rest, ice, crutches with partial weight-bearing.
- Week 2–4: Begin physical therapy. Gentle range of motion and mobility work.
- Week 5–8: Progress to strengthening. Discontinue crutches.
- 2–4 Months: Resume low-impact activities. Running and sports only with clearance.

Preventing Common Complications

Because Nobody Has Time for Blood Clots or Hip Dislocations

Packing Tips, Mental Prep, and All the Weird Stuff Nobody Told You About

1. Blood Clots (DVT/PE)
- Take blood thinners as prescribed
- Do ankle pumps and early walking
- Wear compression socks if recommended

"The scariest part for me was the clot risk," said Melanie, 66. "But staying mobile helped. I walked my hallway every hour."

2. Hip Dislocation
Especially important after posterior approach. Avoid:
- Crossing your legs
- Twisting your torso while feet are planted
- Sitting on low or soft chairs

3. Infection
- Keep incision clean and dry
- No soaking or swimming until cleared
- Watch for fever, chills, or drainage

4. Nerve Injury
Usually temporary, especially with anterior approach (e.g., thigh numbness). Still, report any prolonged numbness, burning, or weakness.

5. Limp or Leg Length Discrepancy
Can occur with muscle weakness or when new joint placement slightly alters leg length. Addressed with rehab or (occasionally) a shoe lift.

Jason M. Aucoin

9

SHOULDER SURGERY – WHAT YOU NEED TO KNOW

Or, "The Joint That Does It All... Until It Doesn't"

Shoulder Complex Anatomy

Like a Marvel Superhero, It's Got Range – But at a Cost

The shoulder is the most mobile joint in the human body—and the least stable. It's more of a complex team than a single joint. Picture it less like a hinge, more like a suspension bridge held together by cables, muscles, and hope.

Key Players:
- Glenohumeral Joint: The main "ball and socket," where the humeral head fits into the glenoid (a shallow cup on the scapula).
- Acromioclavicular (AC) Joint: Where the collarbone meets the highest part of your shoulder blade.
- Scapulothoracic Articulation: Not a true joint, but essential for movement—where the shoulder blade glides along the rib cage.
- Sternoclavicular Joint: Where the clavicle connects to the sternum.

Supporting these are:

- Rotator Cuff Muscles: Supraspinatus, infraspinatus, teres minor, subscapularis—your stabilizers, lifters, and external rotators.
- Labrum: A cartilage ring deepening the glenoid socket.
- Ligaments & Capsule: Tissues keeping the humeral head centered.
- Deltoid & Trapezius: Powerhouses for lifting and reaching.

The trade-off for all that range? The shoulder is prone to wear, tear, and trauma—especially as we age or repeat the same motion (hello, swimmers, pitchers, painters, and desk warriors).

Packing Tips, Mental Prep, and All the Weird Stuff Nobody Told You About

Diagnostic Evaluation of Shoulder Pathologies

When Pain Is More Than Just a "Tweaked Muscle"

Most people ignore shoulder pain until it's impossible to lift a coffee mug or put on a jacket. By the time a doctor evaluates it, you're often dealing with something more serious than overuse.

Common Reasons for Evaluation:
- Persistent pain (especially at night or with overhead activity)
- Weakness or inability to raise the arm
- Instability or frequent dislocations
- Grinding, clicking, or catching
- Pain that doesn't improve with rest or physical therapy

Your Diagnostic Work-Up Might Include:
- X-rays: To check for arthritis, bone spurs, or dislocation.
- MRI or MR Arthrogram: Crucial for seeing the soft tissues—tendons, labrum, cartilage.
- Ultrasound: Real-time imaging of the rotator cuff in motion.
- Physical Exam: Specific strength tests (like empty can, Hawkins-Kennedy, lift-off) to pinpoint the issue.

"I thought I just had bursitis," said Paul, 46. "Turns out I had a full-thickness rotator cuff tear. The MRI told the real story."

Rotator Cuff Procedures

The Shoulder Workhorse That Breaks Down Like an Old Fan Belt

The rotator cuff is a collection of four small but mighty muscles and tendons that keep the shoulder joint centered and rotating smoothly. It's also the most common site of shoulder surgery in adults over 40.

Partial vs. Complete Tears
Partial Tear:
- A frayed or incomplete tear of the tendon.
- May cause pain but not always weakness.
- Often treated non-surgically at first (physical therapy, injections).

Full-Thickness (Complete) Tear:
- Tendon is completely detached from the bone.
- Causes weakness, difficulty lifting the arm.

Can't Bend? Can't Snap? Can't Stop Laughing!

Jason M. Aucoin
- Often surgical—especially if you're under 70 or active.

"I could barely brush my hair," said Lisa, 54. *"My supraspinatus tendon was completely off the bone."*

Size & Shape Matter:
- Small (<1 cm): Often easier to repair, better prognosis.
- Large/Massive (>5 cm): May involve multiple tendons and retraction—more complex repairs or even grafts needed.

Surgical Options and Considerations

1. Arthroscopic Repair
- Minimally invasive: small incisions, camera-guided tools
- Tendon is re-anchored to bone with sutures and anchors
- Less pain, faster healing, fewer complications than open surgery

2. Open Repair
- Larger incision
- Used for larger or retracted tears, revision surgeries
- Allows better access but longer recovery

3. Mini-Open Repair
- Combines both techniques: arthroscopic evaluation + small open incision for repair

4. Tendon Transfers or Grafts
- Used when the tendon is too damaged to reattach
- Another tendon (e.g., latissimus dorsi) may be moved to take over the role

5. Reverse Shoulder Replacement (for massive, irreparable tears + arthritis)
- Ball and socket are reversed so the deltoid muscle can move the arm without the rotator cuff

Key Considerations:
- Age & Activity Level: A younger, active person is more likely to benefit from repair.
- Tear Chronicity: Long-standing tears may cause muscle atrophy and fat infiltration, reducing the success rate.
- Rehabilitation Commitment: Recovery is slow (3–6 months or more) and PT is essential.

"The surgery wasn't the hard part," said Jordan, 62. *"It was the six weeks in a sling and learning how to move my shoulder again."*

Shoulder Instability Procedures
Packing Tips, Mental Prep, and All the Weird Stuff Nobody Told You About

When Your Shoulder Feels Like It's on a Hinge Made of Jello

Instability is often the "younger cousin" to rotator cuff tears. It usually affects younger, athletic patients who've had dislocations or subluxations (partial dislocations), particularly from sports or trauma.

You don't need to be an NFL linebacker to blow out your shoulder—it can happen diving for a volleyball, falling off your bike, or even reaching awkwardly in yoga.

Bankart Repair

The Gold Standard for Anterior Instability

When the shoulder dislocates, especially forward, it often tears the labrum—the rim of cartilage that deepens the socket. A Bankart lesion is when that front portion of the labrum detaches from the bone.

Surgical Fix:
The torn labrum is anchored back to the glenoid (shoulder socket) using suture anchors. This is usually done arthroscopically.

Who It's For:
- Athletes with recurrent anterior shoulder dislocations
- Patients who've failed nonoperative rehab
- People under 30 with their first dislocation (high risk of recurrence)

"I dislocated my shoulder three times before I gave in to surgery," said Evan, 21, a college tennis player. "Bankart repair gave me my game back."

Capsular Shift
Tightening a Loose Joint Capsule

Sometimes the labrum is intact, but the joint capsule (the tissue envelope that holds the shoulder in place) is too loose—either naturally or from repeated dislocations.

Surgical Fix:
Surgeons "shift" or fold and suture the capsule to reduce excess volume and restore tightness—like tailoring an oversized jacket.

Indications:
- Generalized ligamentous laxity
- Multidirectional instability (shoulder slips forward, backward, and downward)

Can't Bend? Can't Snap? Can't Stop Laughing!

Jason M. Aucoin
- Failed previous stabilization procedures

SLAP Lesion Repair Techniques
When the Top of the Labrum Says "Nope"

SLAP = Superior Labrum from Anterior to Posterior
A tear here affects the top of the labrum—where the biceps tendon anchors. Think of it like peeling wallpaper off the top corner.

Causes:
- Overhead athletes (throwers, swimmers)
- Repetitive strain
- Fall on an outstretched arm
- Heavy lifting (especially jerking motions)

Symptoms:
- Deep pain inside the shoulder
- Clicking or catching with movement
- Weakness, especially overhead

Repair Options:
- Debridement: Trim frayed edges (in older, less active patients).
- SLAP Repair: Re-anchor the labrum using sutures.
- Biceps Tenodesis: Detach and re-anchor the biceps tendon lower down to reduce strain (common in patients over 40).

"I couldn't do a single pull-up," said Trevor, 39, an amateur CrossFitter. "Turns out, it wasn't a strength issue—it was a torn SLAP."

Frozen Shoulder Management
Adhesive Capsulitis: The Shoulder's Worst Mood Swing

Frozen shoulder is not a surgical problem—at least not at first. It's a condition where the shoulder capsule tightens and thickens, limiting range of motion and causing pain.

Phases:
1. Freezing (painful loss of motion begins)
2. Frozen (stiffness dominates, pain may decrease)
3. Thawing (motion gradually returns)

Causes:
- Often unknown
- More common in women, diabetics, thyroid disorders
- Can follow trauma or surgery

Treatment:
Packing Tips, Mental Prep, and All the Weird Stuff Nobody Told You About

- Aggressive physical therapy
- Steroid injections
- Oral anti-inflammatories
- Hydrodilatation (joint capsule distention with fluid)
- Rarely: Manipulation under anesthesia or arthroscopic capsular release

"I went from not being able to reach my bra strap to doing yoga again," said Marcy, 52. *"But it took a full year."*

Post-Operative Immobilization Strategies

Why That Sling Is Your Best Friend (and Your Biggest Nuisance)

Depending on the procedure, your surgeon will prescribe specific immobilization protocols—because moving too soon can undo all the repairs.

Standard Guidelines:

- Rotator Cuff Repair:
  Sling with an abduction pillow for 4–6 weeks. Passive motion only at first.

- Bankart or Capsular Shift:
  Sling in internal rotation for 2–4 weeks. Early external rotation often restricted.

- SLAP Repair:
  Limited active biceps use. Gradual return to lifting after 6–8 weeks.

- Frozen Shoulder (Post-Release):
  Active motion encouraged immediately to prevent re-stiffening.

Common Tools:
- Slings (with or without abduction support)
- Ice machines or cold compression
- Shower shields and waterproof dressings
- Sleep wedges (sleeping reclined is often easier)

Progressive Return to Function

From Zipping a Coat to Throwing a Ball

Recovery after shoulder surgery is a slow burn. Unlike hip or knee surgeries, which allow early weight-bearing, the shoulder relies on healing soft tissue and patient dedication to therapy.

Typical Recovery Milestones:
Can't Bend? Can't Snap? Can't Stop Laughing!

Jason M. Aucoin

- 0–6 Weeks: Immobilization, passive motion only
- 6–12 Weeks: Begin active-assisted, then active motion
- 3–4 Months: Strength training begins
- 5–6 Months: Full activity for most patients
- 6–12 Months: Return to overhead sports or heavy labor

"Reaching above my head took four months," said Angela, 45, after a rotator cuff repair. "But now I'm swimming again—and pain-free."

Your shoulder may seem small compared to your hip or knee, but its complexity and recovery demands make it one of the most intricate orthopedic journeys. The key isn't just the surgery—it's the partnership between you, your surgeon, and your physical therapist.

Packing Tips, Mental Prep, and All the Weird Stuff Nobody Told You About

10

Elbow & Wrist Surgery Essentials

The Hinges of Daily Life—Until They Won't Bend (or Stop Hurting)

When people think of joint surgery, they often picture hips or knees. But elbows and wrists—smaller and often overlooked—can be just as life-disrupting when they stop working right. Try brushing your teeth, opening a jar, or shaking someone's hand without a pain-free, flexible elbow or wrist. Spoiler alert: it's not happening.

Elbow Anatomy and Function

Three Bones, One Hinge, Infinite Motion

Your elbow is a marvel of biomechanical engineering, allowing both flexion-extension and rotation of the forearm (supination/pronation).

The Players:
- Humerus (upper arm)
- Ulna (inner forearm bone)
- Radius (outer forearm bone)

Key Structures:
- Ulnar Collateral Ligament (UCL): Stabilizes the inner elbow, especially important in throwing athletes.
  Tendons: Where muscles attach to bone—these often become inflamed or torn.
- Nerves: Especially the ulnar nerve, which wraps around the elbow and can become compressed (cue tingling fingers).
- Joint Capsule & Cartilage: Helps with movement and cushioning.

Can't Bend? Can't Snap? Can't Stop Laughing!

Jason M. Aucoin

Common Elbow Conditions

Tennis Elbow (Lateral Epicondylitis):
- Overuse injury involving the extensor tendons on the outside of the elbow.
- Caused by repetitive gripping or lifting.
- Common in tennis players, but also in office workers, mechanics, and baristas.

Golfer's Elbow (Medial Epicondylitis):
- Involves the flexor tendons on the inside of the elbow.
- Think repetitive wrist flexion or forearm strain.

"I hadn't swung a club in years," joked Carla, 42, a baker. "Turns out kneading dough all day gave me Golfer's Elbow."

Surgical Fix:
Only after failed conservative treatment. Surgery involves removing damaged tendon tissue and reattaching healthy portions. Often done arthroscopically or via small open incision.

UCL Reconstruction (Tommy John Surgery)

A Rite of Passage for Many Baseball Pitchers

Originally performed on Dodgers pitcher Tommy John in 1974, this surgery has saved countless athletic careers.

Who Needs It?
- Mostly overhead throwing athletes—baseball, javelin, football QBs.
- People with chronic inner elbow pain, instability, or a "pop" during a throw.

The Procedure:
- The torn UCL is replaced using a tendon graft (often from the forearm, hamstring, or foot).
- A tunnel is drilled in the humerus and ulna; the graft is weaved through and secured.

"Before surgery, I couldn't throw a ball without pain," said Malik, 19, a collegiate pitcher. "Now I'm throwing harder than ever."

Recovery:
- 12–18 months before returning to competitive throwing.
- Rehab focuses on gradually rebuilding strength, mechanics, and preventing re-injury.

Packing Tips, Mental Prep, and All the Weird Stuff Nobody Told You About

Cubital Tunnel Syndrome Procedures

When the Funny Bone Isn't Funny Anymore

Compression of the ulnar nerve at the elbow—causing numbness, tingling, or weakness in the ring and pinky fingers.

Symptoms:
- Numbness in fingers
- Weak grip
- Difficulty with fine motor tasks
- Pain that worsens with elbow flexion

Surgical Options:
- Ulnar Nerve Decompression: Freeing the nerve from tight tissue.
- Anterior Transposition: Moving the nerve to a less vulnerable position (in front of the elbow).
- Medial Epicondylectomy: Removing part of the bony ridge compressing the nerve.

"It felt like electric shocks down my arm," said Ron, 60. "After the nerve transposition, I got sensation back in my fingers."

Elbow Surgery Recovery Timelines

Patience, Bracing, and Physical Therapy Galore

Recovery varies widely based on the procedure and the patient's occupation or sport. Here's a general breakdown:

Tennis/Golfer's Elbow Release:
- Immobilization: Short (1–2 weeks)
- Return to Light Use: 4–6 weeks
- Return to Sports or Heavy Work: 3–4 months

UCL Reconstruction:
- Immobilization in brace: 1–2 weeks
- Gradual range-of-motion work: Starts around week 2
- Strengthening & Throwing Rehab: 3–6 months
- Return to Sport: 12–18 months

Cubital Tunnel Surgery:
- Sling or splint: 1–2 weeks
- Light activity: 2–4 weeks
- Full use: 6–12 weeks

Can't Bend? Can't Snap? Can't Stop Laughing!

- Nerve recovery: May take months to a year depending on severity

"I had to wear a giant hinged elbow brace for six weeks," said Tara, 34, after UCL surgery. *"At first I hated it—but it taught me how much I use my elbow without realizing it."*

Wrist Anatomy and Biomechanics

Precision Hinges with the Strength of Steel and the Grace of Ballet

Your wrist is not a single joint—it's a complex orchestra of small bones, tendons, nerves, and ligaments that give you the power to write, grip, twist, type, throw, and gesture wildly during arguments. It's a miracle of precision and movement—until it's not.

Carpal Tunnel Release

When the Nerve Gets Squeezed Like a Subway Rider in Rush Hour

The carpal tunnel is a narrow passageway on the palm side of your wrist. It houses the median nerve and several tendons. When the space gets too tight—because of swelling, repetitive strain, or inflammation—the median nerve gets compressed.

Symptoms:
- Numbness and tingling in the thumb, index, and middle fingers
- Pain at night or while using the hand
- Weak grip or tendency to drop objects

"I'd wake up shaking my hand like a thermometer," said Leena, a graphic designer. *"Carpal tunnel was ruining my work—and my sleep."*

Surgical Solution:
- Open Release: Small incision in the palm to cut the ligament compressing the nerve.
- Endoscopic Release: Tiny camera and instruments used through smaller incisions. Less scarring, quicker recovery for some.

Recovery:
- Return to light activity in a few days to a week
- Full recovery and strength in 6–12 weeks
- Relief is often dramatic, especially when caught early

Scaphoid Fractures and TFCC Injuries

Packing Tips, Mental Prep, and All the Weird Stuff Nobody Told You About

The Wrist's Hidden Troublemakers

Scaphoid Fractures:
- The scaphoid is a small bone near the base of the thumb.
- It's notorious for poor blood supply, which makes healing tricky.
- Caused by falls on an outstretched hand.

Symptoms:
- Pain near the base of the thumb
- Swelling that doesn't go away
- Sometimes mistaken for a sprain

Treatment:
- Non-displaced fractures: Cast for 6–12 weeks
- Displaced or non-healing fractures: Surgical screw fixation

"I thought I just sprained it skateboarding," said Jordan, 18. "Six weeks later, it still hurt. Turns out it was fractured—and needed surgery."

TFCC Injuries (Triangular Fibrocartilage Complex):
The TFCC is the shock absorber of the wrist, located on the pinky side. It stabilizes the distal radioulnar joint and helps with rotation.

Causes:
- Falls, twisting injuries
- Overuse in racket sports, gymnastics, or repetitive lifting
- Degeneration with age

Symptoms:
- Pain on the ulnar (pinky) side of the wrist
- Clicking or catching
- Weak grip or wrist instability

Treatment:
- Splinting, injections
- Arthroscopic repair or debridement for persistent cases

Wrist Fusion vs. Arthroplasty

When Mobility is the Price of Pain Relief

When the wrist is severely damaged—often by arthritis, trauma, or failed repairs—patients face two surgical roads:

Can't Bend? Can't Snap? Can't Stop Laughing!

Jason M. Aucoin

Wrist Fusion (Arthrodesis):
- The wrist bones are permanently fused to stop motion and pain.
- Results in loss of wrist mobility, but excellent pain relief and strength.
- Common in manual laborers who prioritize function over flexibility.

Wrist Arthroplasty (Joint Replacement):
- Damaged joint surfaces are replaced with artificial implants.
- Preserves some motion and improves comfort.
- Ideal for low-demand patients, often older adults who need mobility for daily tasks.

"Fusion made my wrist solid—I can swing a hammer again," said Ray, 53, a carpenter. *"I don't miss the movement as much as I thought."*

Specialized Rehabilitation for Hand Function
Hand Therapy is a Whole Profession for a Reason

Rehab after wrist and hand surgery is intensely specialized. This isn't just about regaining strength—it's about fine motor skills, coordination, and nerve recovery.

`Certified Hand Therapists (CHTs):`
Occupational or physical therapists with advanced training in hand, wrist, and elbow rehab.

Goals of Hand Therapy:
- Regain grip strength
- Improve range of motion
- Re-train fine motor tasks like buttoning, typing, writing
- Prevent scar adhesions and stiffness

Tools Used:
- Custom-molded splints
- Putty, balls, and resistance bands
- Mirror therapy for nerve injuries
- Dexterity tools (pegboards, puzzles, sensory kits)

"It felt like kindergarten playtime," laughed Gina, 66, after TFCC surgery. *"But the therapy toys made my hand work again."*

Occupational Considerations for Recovery
Because Not Everyone Sits at a Desk

Returning to work after wrist or elbow surgery depends on your job type, dominant hand, and surgical outcome.

Desk Jobs:
Packing Tips, Mental Prep, and All the Weird Stuff Nobody Told You About

- Can return within days for minor procedures
- May need ergonomic supports (wrist braces, vertical mouse)
- Gradual ramp-up in typing/hand use

Manual Laborers:
- Often out of work for 6–12 weeks or more
- May require retraining if heavy lifting is no longer possible
- Workers' comp and disability plans often factor into planning

Artists, Musicians, Surgeons:
- Recovery is high-stakes and high-stress
- Fine motor precision rehab is essential
- May require longer recovery and psychological support

"As a pianist, I couldn't rush recovery," said Nadia, 37, post-carpal tunnel surgery. "The first time I played a scale pain-free, I cried."

Jason M. Aucoin

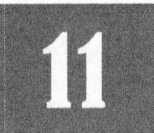

ANKLE & FOOT SURGERIES: STEP-BY-STEP RECOVERY

Because Every Step Matters More Than You Think

The foot and ankle contain 26 bones, 33 joints, and over 100 muscles, tendons, and ligaments. It's an architectural marvel that takes the full force of your body—step after step, mile after mile. But when something goes wrong, even walking across the room can feel like climbing Everest barefoot.

Ankle Joint Anatomy and Mechanics

The Workhorse That Balances Power and Precision

The ankle is a hinge joint, allowing up-and-down movement (dorsiflexion and plantarflexion) and contributing to side-to-side motion via nearby joints.

Major Components:
- Tibia & Fibula: The two leg bones forming the top of the joint
- Talus: The foot bone that receives the weight and distributes it
- Ligaments: Including the ATFL (anterior talofibular ligament) and CFL (calcaneofibular ligament)—key to ankle stability
- Tendons: Most notably, the Achilles tendon
- Subtalar joint: Allows for side-to-side tilting and adaptability to uneven surfaces

"I never thought about my ankle—until it stopped working," said Dylan, a recreational runner. "Turns out it's like the unsung hero of mobility."

Achilles Tendon Procedures

Rupture Repair Techniques

The Snap Heard 'Round the Calf

Packing Tips, Mental Prep, and All the Weird Stuff Nobody Told You About

The Achilles tendon is the largest and strongest tendon in your body, connecting your calf muscles to your heel. But once it tears—often with a loud pop—you're in for a long haul.

Who's at Risk?
- Weekend warriors
- Jumping or pivoting athletes
- Men aged 30–50
- People on certain antibiotics (like fluoroquinolones)

Surgical Repair Options:
- Open Repair: Direct suturing of the tendon ends via a midline incision
- Mini-Open or Percutaneous Repair: Smaller incisions, sometimes using a special jig system
- Augmentation: Using grafts or other tissue for chronic or re-ruptures

"It sounded like someone cracked a whip behind me," recalled Marcus, 41. *"I turned around, but no one was there. It was my Achilles."*

Post-Surgical Management
- Initial Immobilization: 2–3 weeks in a cast or splint
- Transition to Boot: 4–8 weeks in a walking boot with wedges to gradually return foot to neutral
- Physical Therapy: Begins early with gentle range-of-motion exercises
- Full Recovery Timeline: Often 6–12 months to return to full strength and explosive sports

"The hardest part wasn't the surgery," said Lila, a dancer. *"It was trusting my leg again."*

Ankle Instability Surgery
When Your Ankle Rolls Like It's Made of Jello

Chronic ankle sprains can lead to ligament laxity and instability. When bracing and therapy fail, surgery is often the next step.

Common Procedure:
- Broström-Gould Repair: Tightens the stretched-out ATFL and CFL ligaments, often with additional reinforcement (Gould modification)
- Can be done open or arthroscopically

Recovery:
- Non-weight-bearing: 2–3 weeks
- Progressive weight-bearing in boot: Weeks 3–6

Can't Bend? Can't Snap? Can't Stop Laughing!

- PT and balance training: Weeks 6–12
- Return to sports: 3–6 months

"I rolled my ankle so many times, I lost count," said Bree, a high school soccer player. "After surgery, it finally felt solid again."

Ankle Arthroscopy Procedures
Tiny Tools for Big Fixes

Minimally invasive and highly versatile, ankle arthroscopy uses a camera and small tools inserted through tiny incisions to diagnose and treat joint issues.

Used For:
- Removing loose bone or cartilage
- Debriding inflamed tissue
- Fixing osteochondral lesions (cartilage injuries)
- Treating impingement syndromes

Benefits:
- Less pain
- Smaller incisions
- Faster recovery
- Often outpatient

Recovery Timeline:
- Crutches for 1–2 weeks
- Physical therapy by week 2–3
- Return to normal activity in 4–6 weeks (depending on what was treated)

Midfoot and Forefoot Surgery
The Zone of Arches, Balance, and Bunions

The midfoot and forefoot play vital roles in shock absorption, balance, and toe-off propulsion with every step.

Bunion Correction (Hallux Valgus Surgery)
When Your Big Toe Points East, and Your Shoe Won't Fit

A bunion is a bony prominence at the base of the big toe, often painful and progressive.

Surgical Options:
- Osteotomy: Cutting and realigning the bone
- Lapidus Procedure: Fusing the joint at the midfoot
- Minimally Invasive Techniques: Smaller incisions with faster healing

Packing Tips, Mental Prep, and All the Weird Stuff Nobody Told You About

Recovery:
- Protected weight-bearing in a post-op shoe or boot for 4–6 weeks
- Full return to normal footwear around 8–10 weeks
- Swelling may last up to 6 months
- High heels? Usually a no-go post-op

"I just wanted to wear real shoes again," said Joan, 58. *"And not cry halfway through dinner."*

Hammertoe Procedures
Crooked Toes, Straightened Lives

A hammertoe is when a toe bends at the middle joint, often rubbing inside shoes and causing corns or ulcers.

Surgical Fixes:
- Tendon Transfer: Rebalances muscle forces
- Joint Resection or Fusion: Straightens the toe permanently
- Sometimes hardware (pins, screws) is used for alignment

Recovery:
- Walking in a special shoe immediately or after a few days
- Stitches out at 2 weeks
- Full return to shoes in 4–6 weeks

The right surgery, paired with focused recovery, can literally help you find your footing again.

Weight-Bearing Progression Protocols
From Hovering to Heel Strike: Learning to Trust Your Foot Again

After any foot or ankle surgery, weight-bearing isn't just about putting your foot down—it's about timing, trust, and tissues. Recovery hinges (sometimes literally) on how and when you apply pressure to the healing area.

Why Weight-Bearing Matters:
- Promotes circulation and healing
- Stimulates bone remodeling and strength
- Prevents muscle atrophy and joint stiffness

But rush it, and you risk re-injury. Delay too long, and you risk muscle loss and stiffness.

Typical Progression Protocols:

Can't Bend? Can't Snap? Can't Stop Laughing!

Jason M. Aucoin

Phase	Timeframe	Description
Non-Weight-Bearing (NWB)	0–2 weeks	No pressure on the surgical foot; crutches or walker
Toe-Touch or Partial WB	Weeks 2–4	Light foot contact (10–20% of body weight); still with aid
Progressive WB	Weeks 4–6	Gradually increase pressure; transition to walking boot
Full WB in Boot/Shoe	Weeks 6–8	Begin walking without aid; full foot loading
Unrestricted WB	8+ weeks	Back to full mobility; start functional movements

"I thought I was ready to walk without the boot," said Raj, 35, after Achilles surgery. "I tried to carry laundry and ended up right back on the couch for a week. Lesson learned: trust the timeline, not your ego."

Footwear Considerations during Recovery
Forget Fashion—this is a Foot's Healing Wardrobe

Your choice of post-op footwear isn't about style—it's about structure. The right shoe can mean the difference between steady progress and a setback.

Key Features to Look For:
- Stability: Wide base, rigid soles to limit motion
- Support: Good arch and heel counter
- Cushioning: Helps absorb impact
- Easy Entry: Velcro or elastic if mobility is limited

Shoe Types Based on Recovery Stage:
- Post-Op Shoes (Weeks 0–4): Flat, rigid soles to prevent toe-off
- Walking Boots (Weeks 4–6): Removable, with rocker bottom to simulate gait
- Transition Shoes (Weeks 6–8): Supportive sneakers, often with inserts
- Final Phase (8+ Weeks): Regular shoes, often custom-fitted or orthopedic

"I called them my 'Frankenstein boots'—big, clunky, and life-saving," joked Miriam, 64. "I didn't win any fashion awards, but I also didn't fall."

Orthotics May Be Prescribed:
- Especially for arch support or correcting gait abnormalities post-surgery
- Custom orthotics help redistribute weight and prevent compensatory injuries

Return to Walking, Running and Sports
From Shuffle to Stride: Reclaiming Your Motion
Packing Tips, Mental Prep, and All the Weird Stuff Nobody Told You About

Getting back to walking, jogging, or sports isn't just about strength—it's about confidence, control, and coordination.

General Timeline (Varies by Procedure & Patient):

Activity	Typical Return Window
Walking (Unaided)	6–8 weeks
Treadmill/Light Cardio	10–12 weeks
Running (Short Distance)	4–6 months
Sport-Specific Drills	5–7 months
Full Sport Return	6–12 months

Keys to Success:
- Structured Physical Therapy: Focus on strength, proprioception, and balance
- Gait Analysis: Ensure proper mechanics before impact exercises
- Gradual Progression: Introduce agility and pivoting slowly

"The first time I jogged again, I teared up," said Don, a retired firefighter. "It wasn't fast or graceful, but it was mine."

Warning Signs to Watch For:
- Pain that worsens after activity
- Swelling that doesn't subside overnight
- Limping or altered gait
- Catching, locking, or instability in the joint

Jason M. Aucoin

12

SPINAL JOINT SURGERIES

The Backbone of Mobility—And What Happens When It Needs a Tune-Up

Spinal surgeries are often painted as terrifying last resorts. But let's be honest—when your spine is screaming, and conservative treatments are no longer cutting it, the idea of reclaiming pain-free movement is more than just appealing—it's necessary. This chapter walks through spinal surgeries in the neck (cervical), mid-back (thoracic), and lower back (lumbar), breaking down the procedures, recovery, and real-life patient experiences along the way.

Cervical Spine Procedures

Your Neck's Not Just Holding Your Head Up—It's Doing Precision Engineering

The cervical spine—those top seven vertebrae from C1 to C7—is a highway for nerves and responsible for head movement, balance, and sensation in your arms. When degenerative changes, herniated discs, or trauma disrupt this system, surgery may be on the table.

Disc Replacement vs. Fusion
Motion Saver or Stability Provider?

Anterior Cervical Discectomy and Fusion (ACDF) is the most common neck surgery. Surgeons remove the damaged disc through the front of the neck and fuse the adjacent vertebrae with bone grafts and hardware.

- Pros: Time-tested, high success rates
- Cons: Limits motion at that spinal level, can stress adjacent discs over time

Cervical Disc Replacement (CDR) is the newer, motion-preserving option. The disc is removed and replaced with an artificial disc.

Packing Tips, Mental Prep, and All the Weird Stuff Nobody Told You About

- Pros: Maintains motion, quicker recovery, less adjacent segment stress
- Cons: Not ideal for all patients (e.g., those with severe arthritis)

"I went with a disc replacement because I'm a drummer," said Vic, 42. *"I needed my neck to move freely—and it does."*

Post-Operative Mobility Concerns

You'll likely wear a neck brace for 1–3 weeks, avoid lifting, and limit screen time (goodbye, Netflix marathons—temporarily). Physical therapy focuses on gentle range-of-motion exercises, posture correction, and nerve glides.

Full recovery: 6–12 weeks, though some patients feel dramatically better within days.

Thoracic Spine Considerations

The Most Stable Part of Your Spine—But Not Immune to Trouble

The thoracic spine (T1–T12) is your ribcage's structural partner and is rarely the star of spine surgery shows. But when it does need intervention—think herniated discs, scoliosis, or tumors—it's complex.

Challenges:
- Access is difficult due to rib and lung proximity
- Surgery often involves posterior or lateral approaches, and sometimes robotic guidance
- Recovery is longer and may include hospital stays of 4–7 days

Procedures:
- Discectomy or decompression for herniations
- Spinal fusion for scoliosis or kyphosis
- Tumor resection with reconstruction, if needed

"I had scoliosis correction at 29," shared Ana. *"The hardest part wasn't the pain—it was learning how to trust my back again."*

Lumbar Procedures and Recovery

When Your Low Back Isn't Backing You Up Anymore

Can't Bend? Can't Snap? Can't Stop Laughing!

Jason M. Aucoin

The lumbar spine—your lower back—is a common pain hotspot. Between poor posture, sitting jobs, lifting toddlers, and forgotten gym form, it's under constant pressure.

Microdiscectomy
A Tiny Cut That Makes a Huge Difference

Used for herniated discs pressing on spinal nerves (often causing leg pain), this is a minimally invasive surgery.

- Procedure: Surgeon removes the herniated portion through a small incision
- Hospital stay: Often outpatient or 1 night
- Recovery: Walk the same day; return to light work in 2 weeks; full activity in 6–8 weeks

"The sciatica disappeared almost instantly," said Jordan, 36. *"It felt like someone flipped a switch."*

Laminectomy
Opening the Door for Nerve Relief

Used to treat spinal stenosis, this surgery removes part of the lamina (the roof of the spinal canal) to relieve nerve compression.

- Often done in older adults with chronic back/leg pain
- May be combined with fusion if instability is present
- Recovery is longer than microdiscectomy: 6–12 weeks

Spinal Fusion Techniques
When Stability Becomes the Priority

Fusion involves connecting two or more vertebrae using rods, screws, and bone grafts. Common in:

- Degenerative disc disease
- Spondylolisthesis
- Failed prior surgeries

Techniques:
- PLIF (Posterior Lumbar Interbody Fusion)
- TLIF (Transforaminal Lumbar Interbody Fusion)
- ALIF (Anterior Lumbar Interbody Fusion)—from the front

Recovery:

Packing Tips, Mental Prep, and All the Weird Stuff Nobody Told You About

- Hospital stay: 2–5 days
- Brace may be required
- Physical therapy begins after initial healing
- Return to full activity: 3–6 months

"Fusion scared me, but after years of instability, I finally feel like I can move without flinching," said Darnell, 53.

Minimally Invasive Spine Surgery (MISS)

Small Incisions, Big Gains?

Minimally Invasive Spine Surgery (MISS) is the sleek, high-tech cousin of traditional spine surgery—and its goal is simple: achieve the same results with less tissue disruption.

Rather than making a large incision and moving muscles aside, surgeons use tubular retractors, microscopes, and sometimes robotic assistance to access the spine through a much smaller opening.

Common MISS Procedures:
- Microdiscectomy
- Spinal decompression (laminotomy)
- Spinal fusions (using percutaneous screws)

Benefits:
- Shorter hospital stays (often outpatient)
- Less postoperative pain
- Lower risk of infection
- Faster return to daily life

Limitations:
- Not suitable for complex spinal deformities or multi-level fusions
- Requires experienced surgeons and advanced equipment
- May take longer to perform (but saves time in recovery)

"I walked out of the hospital the same day," said Lena, 45, after a minimally invasive TLIF. *"It felt almost surreal—like spine surgery wasn't supposed to be that gentle."*

Recovery Positioning and Movement Restrictions

Healing Is a Full-Time Job—and Your Body Has Rules

Can't Bend? Can't Snap? Can't Stop Laughing!

Jason M. Aucoin

Your spine is like a stack of books: misalign one, and the whole structure shifts. Post-surgery, maintaining alignment is critical.

Positioning Guidelines:
- No twisting or bending for several weeks
- Use the log roll technique to get in and out of bed
- Sleep on your back or side with a pillow between your knees
- Use firm mattresses and recliners that support lumbar curves

Movement Restrictions:
- No lifting more than 5–10 pounds initially
- Avoid sitting for long periods—walk frequently, but in short bursts
- Use a grabber tool—no bending to tie shoes or pick up dropped items
- Driving? Only after being cleared by your surgeon and stopping narcotics

"The grabber was my MVP," joked Kevin, 60, post-fusion. "I even used it to change the TV channel once—true story."

Brace or No Brace?
Some patients are issued lumbar or cervical braces to limit motion and stabilize healing. Follow instructions strictly—overuse can lead to muscle atrophy, while underuse may delay healing.

Long-Term Spine Health Maintenance

What Comes After Recovery? Prevention.

Once you've invested in your spine, you don't want to undo that progress. Long-term health is all about protecting, strengthening, and respecting your back.

Post-Rehab Exercise:
- Focus on core strengthening: planks, bridges, bird-dogs
- Engage in low-impact cardio: swimming, elliptical, walking
- Incorporate stretching and mobility work to keep tissue pliable

"Pilates saved me," said Priya, 39, who had a lumbar microdiscectomy. "I felt my posture improve, and my back just... held itself better."

Lifestyle Adjustments:
- Ergonomics matter: invest in proper chairs, monitor setups, and lumbar supports
- Weight management: excess weight stresses spinal joints
- Quit smoking: it reduces blood flow and delays healing
- Hydration and nutrition: discs thrive on fluid and proper nutrients

Mental Health Counts, Too:

Packing Tips, Mental Prep, and All the Weird Stuff Nobody Told You About

Spine surgery recovery can be isolating and slow. Depression and anxiety are not uncommon. Stay connected, talk to a therapist if needed, and celebrate every small win—even tying your shoes solo again is a milestone.

A Word from the Front Lines:

"It's not just about fixing something—it's about teaching your body and brain how to live differently," said Dr. Neeta Ghosh, a spine surgeon and yoga advocate. *"Surgery gets you out of crisis, but lifestyle keeps you out of the ER."*

Jason M. Aucoin

13

SMALL JOINT SURGERIES: FINGERS & TOES

Tiny Joints, Big Impact: When the Smallest Surgeries Mean the Most

The joints in your fingers and toes may be small, but anyone who has experienced stiffness, pain, or deformity in these areas knows—they hold an outsized role in our daily lives. Whether you're buttoning a shirt, texting, typing, or just walking across the room, these tiny hinges work hard. When injury, arthritis, or disease impairs them, surgery may be necessary to restore form and function.

Anatomy of Digital Joints

In each finger, there are three joints (except the thumb, which has two):
- DIP (Distal Interphalangeal) – closest to the nail
- PIP (Proximal Interphalangeal) – middle joint
- MCP (Metacarpophalangeal) – where the finger meets the hand

Each toe similarly has tiny joints with less mobility but significant structural responsibility. They're supported by ligaments, tendons, synovial sheaths, and—critically—digital nerves that make sensation incredibly precise.

Trigger Finger Release

When Your Finger's "Click" Is No Longer Cute

Trigger finger, or stenosing tenosynovitis, occurs when the flexor tendon becomes irritated and can't glide smoothly through its sheath. The result? A painful popping or locking of the finger when trying to straighten it.

Packing Tips, Mental Prep, and All the Weird Stuff Nobody Told You About

Surgical Release:
- A quick outpatient procedure
- A tiny incision in the palm allows the surgeon to release the sheath
- Sometimes done with local anesthesia only

"The weirdest part? I could instantly open my hand," said Jeanette, 58. "No snap, no catch. Just... smooth."

Recovery:
- Soreness for a few days
- Light activity after a week
- Full use by 2–3 weeks, with hand therapy if stiffness lingers

Dupuytren's Contracture Procedures

When Cords of Tissue Turn Into Cages

Dupuytren's is a genetic condition where the fascia under the skin of the palm thickens into cords, pulling fingers into a bent position. Surgery is often needed when function is significantly impaired.

Options:
- Needle Aponeurotomy: Less invasive, faster recovery, higher recurrence
- Open Fasciectomy: Larger incision, more thorough removal
- Collagenase Injection: Enzyme breaks cords, followed by manual rupture

"I was amazed how my finger straightened after the injection," said Tom, 66. "But I had to stretch it constantly afterward to keep it that way."

Post-Surgical Therapy:
Splinting, stretching, and scar massage are essential to maintaining extension and preventing recurrence.

Digital Joint Replacement Options

Yes, You Can Get a New Finger Joint

For patients with severe arthritis, joint destruction, or post-traumatic degeneration, digital joint replacement (arthroplasty) is an option—though it's not as common as in knees or hips.

Implants:
- Silicone spacers are the most common
- Newer options include metal-polymer or pyrocarbon implants

Can't Bend? Can't Snap? Can't Stop Laughing!

Jason M. Aucoin
- Ideal for MCP and PIP joints, especially in the index and middle fingers

"I was a painter—literally couldn't hold a brush," said Arturo, 70. "The implant gave me enough flexion to start working again."

Recovery:
- Protected movement starts within a week
- Hand therapy is a must
- Full function can take 3–6 months

Post-Operative Hand Therapy

Where the Real Healing Happens

Hand therapy is non-negotiable for finger surgery. Why? Because scar tissue, swelling, and immobility can destroy surgical gains.

Core Elements:
- Range-of-motion exercises within days post-op
- Edema management (compression gloves, elevation)
- Splinting to protect or stretch, depending on surgery type
- Strengthening and fine motor retraining (hello, therapy putty)

"I played piano through therapy," said Marta, 52, post-MCP arthroplasty. "It wasn't pretty at first—but my hand came back."

Digital Nerve Considerations

Cut Here, Lose Feeling There

Surgery on fingers and toes risks damaging the digital nerves, which can lead to:

- Numbness
- Tingling or burning (neuropathy)
- Neuroma formation (painful nerve knot)

Surgeons use loupes (magnifying glasses) and delicate dissection to protect nerves. Still, temporary nerve symptoms are common.

"It felt like ants in my fingertip for two months," said Josh, 38, post trigger release. "But it faded completely."

Packing Tips, Mental Prep, and All the Weird Stuff Nobody Told You About

14

JOINT REPLACEMENTS VS. ARTHROSCOPIES

Understanding the "Fix" Before the First Incision

For many patients facing joint surgery, one of the biggest questions is: "What kind of procedure do I actually need?" The options often boil down to two categories: arthroscopy, a minimally invasive "clean-up" or repair, and joint replacement, a much more involved surgery that replaces worn-out components with artificial ones. They're not interchangeable—but they're often confused.

Decision-Making Process for Procedure Selection

Clarity Comes from Diagnosis, Imaging, and Lifestyle

The choice between arthroscopy and joint replacement isn't just a matter of preference. It depends on:

- The severity of damage:
Arthroscopy is best for mild-to-moderate injuries, like a torn meniscus or a loose cartilage flap. Joint replacement is for severe arthritis or bone-on-bone degeneration.

- Your age and activity level:
Younger patients often start with arthroscopy to delay replacement. Older or less active patients might benefit more from going straight to a joint replacement.

- Patient goals:
Some want to return to high-impact sports; others want to walk without pain. Those goals guide the plan.

Can't Bend? Can't Snap? Can't Stop Laughing!

- Imaging and response to conservative care:
If MRIs show extensive damage and injections or therapy haven't helped, replacement may be inevitable.

"I'd been getting cortisone shots in my knee for years," said Monica, 62. "But once I couldn't walk the grocery aisle without pain, my surgeon said we were past the 'scope-it' stage."

Comparative Recovery Timelines

Arthroscopy = Quick Fix (Sometimes). Replacement = Long Haul

Factor	Arthroscopy	Joint Replacement
Invasiveness	Minimally invasive (tiny incisions)	Major open surgery
Pain Level	Mild-to-moderate	Moderate-to-severe early on
Initial Recovery	1–2 weeks for daily activities	4–6 weeks with assistance
Full Return to Activity	6–8 weeks (depends on joint)	3–6 months
Physical Therapy	Often needed, but shorter	Critical, long-term

"I was walking the next day after my hip arthroscopy," said Jared, 28. "But my dad's knee replacement had him using a walker for two weeks."

Important Note:
Arthroscopy might not solve the problem—it's often diagnostic or palliative. Joint replacements aim for a long-term solution.

Implant Types and Materials

Titanium, Ceramic, Polyethylene—A Joint Buffet

Traditional vs. Robot-Assisted Replacements
Traditional replacements are still common and highly effective, but robot-assisted techniques (like MAKO or ROSA systems) are gaining ground.

- Traditional:
Surgeon uses visual/tactile landmarks for alignment and placement
Pros: Proven track record, lower cost
Cons: Slightly higher variability in outcomes

Packing Tips, Mental Prep, and All the Weird Stuff Nobody Told You About

- Robot-Assisted:
  Real-time 3D mapping, precision cuts, improved alignment
  Pros: Potential for quicker recovery, better joint longevity
  Cons: More expensive, longer OR time, not available everywhere

"With the robot, my surgeon said it was like putting a puzzle together with a laser instead of a blindfold," laughed Mike, 55.

Partial vs. Total Joint Replacements

Sometimes only part of the joint is damaged—meaning a partial replacement could suffice.

- Partial (Unicompartmental):
  Only one side or part of the joint is replaced
  Pros: Smaller incision, faster recovery, retains more natural bone
  Cons: Not suitable for widespread arthritis
  Common in knees and some finger joints

- Total Replacement:
  Entire joint surface is replaced with artificial components
  Pros: Comprehensive solution for severe degeneration
  Cons: Longer recovery, risk of loosening or wear over time

"My partial knee replacement was so easy, I was gardening in three weeks," said Nina, 60. "But my brother had a total one—whole different ballgame."

The right procedure isn't always the one that sounds the easiest or has the quickest recovery—it's the one that fits your joint, lifestyle, and long-term health. Don't be afraid to ask your surgeon why they're recommending one option over another, and don't be shy about second opinions.

Because when it comes to joint surgery, understanding the why is just as important as the how.

Age and Activity Level Considerations

From Marathoners to Mall Walkers—One Size Doesn't Fit All

Age and lifestyle are key factors in determining not just which procedure you get, but when you get it.

- Younger Patients (Under 50):

Surgeons tend to be conservative with replacements. The goal is to preserve the joint for as long as possible using arthroscopy, injections, and physical therapy. This is partly because:
- Replacements wear out over time
- Multiple revisions are riskier and less successful
- Younger patients are typically more active, accelerating wear

"I was 38 when I tore my ACL," recalled Martin. "My surgeon said we'd repair it arthroscopically now, but a replacement may be in my future."

- Middle-Aged Patients (50–65):
This group often sits at the crossroads between repair and replacement. Decision-making is individualized:
  - High-impact athletes may delay replacement
  - Less active individuals may benefit from early intervention

- Older Adults (65+):
If imaging shows severe arthritis, and the goal is to regain mobility with less pain, replacement may be the first choice. Today's implants often last decades, and older patients typically aren't as rough on them.

Longevity of Results and Revision Surgery

Will This Last Forever? Maybe. Maybe Not.

- Arthroscopy Longevity:
Depends on the issue being treated. Meniscus repairs or debridement may buy time, but arthroscopy is rarely curative for advanced arthritis. Many patients eventually require a replacement.

- Joint Replacement Lifespan:
Today's implants last 15–25 years, depending on:
  - Activity level
  - Implant type/material
  - Surgical technique
  - Patient weight and bone health

- Revision Surgery:
When a joint replacement fails due to wear, infection, or loosening, revision surgery is needed. These procedures are:
  - Longer and more complex
  - Often require specialized surgeons
  - May have a longer recovery and more modest outcomes

"My hip replacement lasted 20 years," said Helen, 78. "But the revision wasn't a walk in the park. Still, I'm grateful I got all those years without pain."

Packing Tips, Mental Prep, and All the Weird Stuff Nobody Told You About

Cross-Joint Rehabilitation Principles

Shoulders, Knees, Toes—They All Need TLC

No matter the joint, rehabilitation shares key principles:

- Early Movement:
Prevents stiffness and improves circulation. Some protocols start within 24 hours.

- Pain Management:
Movement hurts—but so does doing nothing. Balancing comfort with progress is critical.

- Progressive Load Bearing:
Whether it's partial weight-bearing on a new ankle or gradually regaining grip strength in your wrist, loading is progressive and guided by your PT.

- Consistency Over Intensity:
The best outcomes come from daily, consistent work, not occasional, high-effort bursts.

- Patient Education:
Knowing what to expect can reduce fear, improve motivation, and encourage independence.

"The rehab after my shoulder replacement was intense," said Joe, 65. *"But I got there by treating it like a part-time job."*

Life After Joint Surgery: Managing Expectations

Reality Check: It's Better, Not Perfect

It's tempting to expect a return to your 20s, but joint surgery aims for relief and function—not immortality.

What You Can Expect:
- Less pain (often dramatically so)
- Improved range of motion
- Easier daily movement (walking, stairs, dressing)
- Return to low-impact activities (swimming, biking, and golfing)

What You Probably Can't Expect:
- High-impact sports (running, skiing, contact sports)

Can't Bend? Can't Snap? Can't Stop Laughing!

Jason M. Aucoin
- Zero limitations
- "Feeling normal" overnight

"My knee doesn't feel exactly like my own," said Lou, 70. "But I can hike again. I'll take that win every time."

Mental Adjustment Matters:

Recovery can be lonely, frustrating, and slower than expected. Some people experience post-op depression or anxiety—especially if they expected a miracle fix. Others are surprised by how much work recovery really is.

But for the vast majority, life is better after joint surgery. Pain is down, movement is up, and the fear of "when will this flare up again?" starts to fade into the background.

Packing Tips, Mental Prep, and All the Weird Stuff Nobody Told You About

15

Pediatric Joint Surgery Considerations

Small Joints, Big Decisions: What Makes Kids Different

When you think of joint surgery, you probably picture adults—older runners with worn-out knees or active teens with torn ACLs. But joint surgery in kids is its own world, filled with unique challenges, enormous emotional stakes, and a lot of courage from tiny patients and their families.

While the fundamentals of joint anatomy and recovery apply to all ages, the developing musculoskeletal system, the presence of growth plates, and the psychological and emotional needs of children make pediatric joint surgery a specialized field requiring thoughtful nuance.

Growth Plate Concerns and Approaches

Why Surgeons Sweat the Small Stuff

In kids, growth isn't just a stage—it's an active process happening in the bone. The growth plates (also called epiphyseal plates) are areas of developing cartilage tissue near the ends of long bones. They're responsible for the bone's length and shape.

The Dilemma:
Any surgical intervention near a growth plate comes with risks:
  Premature closure of the plate
- Uneven limb length
- Angular deformities
- Long-term functional consequences

Can't Bend? Can't Snap? Can't Stop Laughing!

Surgeons trained in pediatric orthopedics use growth-sparing techniques and may delay surgery if possible until the plate has matured.

"My son needed ACL reconstruction at 13," said Heather, mother of a young athlete. *"They used a technique that avoided the growth plate entirely. We were so relieved."*

Congenital Joint Abnormalities

Born Different—And Built Strong

Some children need joint surgery not because of injury, but because of how they were born.

Common congenital joint conditions include:
- Developmental Dysplasia of the Hip (DDH): Hip socket doesn't fully cover the femoral head.
- Clubfoot: Foot is twisted out of shape or position.
- Radial Club Hand: A rare defect where the radius bone is underdeveloped or absent.
- Juvenile Rheumatoid Arthritis (JRA): An autoimmune condition that can affect joint development.

These cases often require a team approach: pediatric orthopedic surgeons, physical therapists, occupational therapists, and sometimes geneticists or neurologists.

Treatment Goals:
- Maximize function
- Support normal development
- Minimize the need for repeated interventions

Developmental Milestones in Recovery

When Healing Collides with Growth

Unlike adults, kids are developing basic skills as they recover. A toddler healing from a hip procedure may be relearning to crawl or walk. A teen may be working to regain confidence in sports or social activity.

"After her surgery, Ella had to learn to walk again—but she also had to keep up with second grade," her dad explained. *"Recovery wasn't just physical; it was emotional and academic."*

Rehab in children often includes:

Packing Tips, Mental Prep, and All the Weird Stuff Nobody Told You About

- Play-based therapy
- Child-specific milestones (e.g., jumping, climbing stairs, playground activities)
- Adaptive equipment that allows freedom while protecting healing joints

Family-Centered Recovery Support

Healing the Whole Household

When a child undergoes surgery, the entire family is affected. Parents become caregivers, therapists, and emotional anchors. Siblings may feel left out or confused. Daily life becomes a mix of medical appointments, school adjustments, and lots of questions.

Hospitals specializing in pediatric care often emphasize family-centered support:
- Child life specialists to help kids process fear and pain
- Parental training in post-op care
- Support groups or peer mentors
- Emotional health resources for both child and parent

"We were trained on how to handle her brace, her meds, even how to talk about pain in ways she understood," said Sara, mother of a 5-year-old with hip dysplasia. *"We didn't feel alone."*

School and Activity Reintegration

Backpacks, Sports, and Peer Questions

Returning to school after joint surgery is more than showing up—it's reintegrating into a world that may not understand what just happened.

Common Challenges:
- Physical limitations (mobility, fatigue, seating)
- Emotional hurdles (feeling "different" or being asked invasive questions)
- Academic delays from missed school

Schools often provide:
- Individualized Education Plans (IEPs) or 504 accommodations
- Modified gym activities
- Extra time for mobility between classes

Returning to sports—if allowed—is usually gradual and supervised. The goal isn't just performance, but confidence and body awareness.

"I missed a whole soccer season," said Sam, age 12. *"But my coach said, 'Let's make next season your comeback.' That meant everything*

Can't Bend? Can't Snap? Can't Stop Laughing!

Jason M. Aucoin

Packing Tips, Mental Prep, and All the Weird Stuff Nobody Told You About

16

Geriatric Joint Surgery Considerations

When Wisdom Meets Wear and Tear: Joint Surgery in the Golden Years

There's a certain grace that comes with aging—wisdom lines on the face, a calm sense of perspective, and, yes, sometimes creaky joints that finally demand a little surgical help. Geriatric joint surgery is rising rapidly, with joint replacements among the most common procedures in older adults. But make no mistake: seniors aren't just "older adults" in surgical planning. They're complex, resilient, and require unique care.

Preoperative Risk Assessment

Looking at the Whole Picture, Not Just the Joint

The first major difference in older adults? Risk profiles. Seniors often present with more than just a knee or hip problem. They have decades of health history behind them—some of it well-managed, some of it lurking quietly in the background.

Comprehensive pre-op evaluation includes:
- Cardiac clearance (older adults are more prone to silent heart disease)
- Pulmonary function checks (especially in smokers or those with COPD)
- Cognitive screening (to gauge risk of post-op delirium)
- Frailty assessments (muscle mass, gait speed, energy levels)

"My surgeon said he was less worried about my arthritis and more about how well my lungs would handle anesthesia," said George, 74, who had a hip replacement last year.

Can't Bend? Can't Snap? Can't Stop Laughing!

Jason M. Aucoin

This evaluation isn't to disqualify—it's to customize and protect.

Medication Management Concerns

When Your Pillbox Looks Like a Pharmacy

Polypharmacy—taking multiple medications—is nearly universal in the senior population. That means a careful medication review is not optional before surgery.

Key concerns:
- Blood thinners: Common for heart disease or stroke prevention, but risky for surgery.
- Diabetes meds: Must be adjusted around fasting, stress, and reduced mobility.
- Pain meds: Seniors are more sensitive to opioids, and are at higher risk for confusion or falls.

Your healthcare team may coordinate with a geriatric pharmacist or primary care physician to fine-tune meds for safety.

Comorbidity Considerations

When Surgery Happens in a Complex Ecosystem

Older patients may have:
- Diabetes
- Hypertension
- Osteoporosis
- Dementia
- Kidney or liver impairment

Each of these conditions affects how the body tolerates anesthesia, metabolizes drugs, and recovers from surgical trauma. The key is collaborative care.

Hospitals may assign:
- A geriatric consult team
- Nutritionists
- Wound care specialists
- Physical and occupational therapists who specialize in elder care

"It wasn't just my knee," said Clara, 82. "They looked at my bones, my heart, even how I walk. It made me feel safer."

Modified Rehabilitation Approaches

Packing Tips, Mental Prep, and All the Weird Stuff Nobody Told You About

Healing Slowly, Steadily, and Safely

Geriatric rehabilitation focuses on function, not just fitness.

That means:
- Gentler progression timelines
- Emphasis on ADLs (activities of daily living)
- Customized therapy to avoid overexertion
- Addressing cognitive fatigue and depression, which can impact motivation

Assistive devices (walkers, canes, grab bars) are often introduced early, not as a crutch, but as freedom tools.

"I hated the walker at first," said Edna, 79. "But it helped me stay independent while I healed."

Fall Prevention during Recovery

Avoiding the Most Dangerous Post-Op Complication

Falls are the number one enemy during geriatric recovery. A single misstep can mean a cascade of injuries, re-hospitalization, and loss of independence.

Prevention strategies include:
- Home safety evaluations (removing rugs, adding nightlights, installing rails)
- Non-slip socks and shoes
- Physical therapy focused on balance and proprioception
- Vision and hearing checks (often overlooked contributors to falls)

Some hospitals offer fall-prevention boot camps for families and caregivers before discharge.

Long-Term Care Planning

Because Recovery Doesn't Always End at 6 Weeks

Sometimes, despite the best plans, recovery is prolonged. A geriatric patient may need:
- A short stay in a rehab facility
- In-home nursing or physical therapy
- Long-term mobility aids or personal care assistance
- Changes in living arrangements (e.g., moving to a single-level home or assisted living)

Can't Bend? Can't Snap? Can't Stop Laughing!

Jason M. Aucoin
This isn't failure—it's adaptation, and planning early makes it empowering.

"We knew my dad wouldn't bounce back like he did at 60," said Linda, whose 88-year-old father had a shoulder replacement. "So we made a plan, and that plan gave us peace."

Packing Tips, Mental Prep, and All the Weird Stuff Nobody Told You About

17

Multi-Joint Considerations and Complex Cases

When It's Not Just One Joint—And Recovery Is a Jigsaw Puzzle

If a single joint surgery is a carefully planned mission, multi-joint surgery or complex reconstruction is a full-blown expedition. It demands strategy, stamina, and synchronization—often across disciplines, surgeons, and stages of recovery.

Rheumatoid Arthritis Surgical Management

When the Immune System Wages War on Your Joints

Rheumatoid arthritis (RA) is the equal-opportunity disabler—affecting knees, hips, shoulders, wrists, even small finger joints. It doesn't play fair, and its unpredictability makes surgical planning extra challenging.

Key considerations include:
- Timing: RA flares can disrupt post-op healing; optimal windows for surgery must be chosen carefully.
- Medication management: Biologics and immunosuppressants like methotrexate may be paused before surgery to reduce infection risk—but pausing can cause disease flare.
- Joint prioritization: Often, multiple joints need surgery. Surgeons will assess which joint's dysfunction is most impairing your function and start there.

"My hands, knees, and shoulders were all affected," said Joelle, 52, living with RA for two decades. *"We had to make a roadmap with my rheumatologist and surgeon working together."*

Staged vs. Simultaneous Bilateral Procedures

Can't Bend? Can't Snap? Can't Stop Laughing!

Jason M. Aucoin
Two Joints, One Trip to the OR—or Two?

Some patients need both knees, both hips, and both shoulders replaced. The question then becomes: do it all at once, or in stages?

Simultaneous surgeries:
- One anesthesia session
- One hospital stay
- Faster overall recovery timeline
- Greater early discomfort and immobility risks

Staged surgeries:
- Less strain on heart, lungs, and rehab capacity
- Allows the first joint to heal before stressing the second
- Ideal for elderly or medically complex patients

"I had both knees done, six months apart," said Reggie, 67. *"It gave me time to rebuild my strength and confidence between."*

This decision is deeply personal—and medical. Some hospitals offer bilateral surgery pathways for healthy, younger patients under age 70 with minimal comorbidities.

Post-Traumatic Reconstruction Challenges

When the Injury Was Years Ago—but you're still paying the Price

Trauma changes everything. A shattered knee from a car accident, a malunioned ankle fracture, or a dislocated shoulder from a fall years ago can leave residual damage, scar tissue, and biomechanical chaos.

Post-traumatic reconstruction is like surgery with a history—it must work around:
- Previous hardware
- Soft tissue damage and adhesions
- Altered anatomy and bone alignment
- Emotional trauma and fear from the original injury

Surgeons often use 3D planning, custom implants, and longer OR times. Recovery tends to be slower, but the functional improvements can be dramatic.

"After my accident, I thought I'd never walk properly again," said Amir, 45. *"The reconstruction gave me a second shot."*

Coordinating Care across Multiple Joints

Packing Tips, Mental Prep, and All the Weird Stuff Nobody Told You About

The Art and Science of Surgical Choreography

When multiple joints are involved—either simultaneously or in sequence—it takes a village of providers to pull off a safe, successful recovery. You may have:
- Multiple orthopedic specialists
- A rheumatologist
- Pain management teams
- Specialized rehab therapists
- A case manager or surgical navigator

A care coordinator or patient advocate becomes essential. They ensure:
- Appointments are synchronized
- Medications don't clash
- Home recovery setups are appropriate for more than one joint
- The patient is emotionally supported through a longer and more complex journey

Quality of Life Improvements and Measurement

Defining Success When It's Not Just One Problem Fixed

When multiple joints are involved, success isn't just about how far you can bend your knee—it's about how your life changes.

Common outcomes patients report:
- Ability to sleep without pain again
- Reduced reliance on walkers or canes
- Returning to hobbies or work
- Less fatigue from overcompensating with "stronger" joints

Surgeons and researchers increasingly use quality of life metrics, like:
- The WOMAC scale (for joint stiffness, function, and pain)
- The SF-36 (a broad health status questionnaire)
- Patient-Reported Outcome Measures (PROMs)

These tools reflect that healing is not just about the body—it's about the whole you.

Can't Bend? Can't Snap? Can't Stop Laughing!

Jason M. Aucoin

PART THREE
POST-OP REALITY

Packing Tips, Mental Prep, and All the Weird Stuff Nobody Told You About

18

PAIN MANAGEMENT (REAL TALK)

The Battle You Weren't Expecting to Fight This Hard

Let's not sugarcoat it: pain after joint surgery is real, and managing it is as much a mental game as a medical one. Whether you're waking up from surgery or two weeks into recovery wondering why your knee still feels like a cement block—this chapter is here to help you understand what's happening, what's normal, and what's not. We'll cover everything from meds to mental strength, cold packs to compression wraps, and throw in some truth from patients who've lived it.

Understanding Post-Surgical Pain

Acute vs. Chronic Pain Patterns

Pain after surgery isn't one-size-fits-all. Immediately post-op, you'll deal with acute pain, which is your body's way of saying: "Hey, we've been through something major!" This pain is expected to decrease steadily over days and weeks.

But sometimes, pain sticks around long after the stitches dissolve. That's chronic post-surgical pain (CPSP), and it can stem from nerve irritation, scar tissue, or inflammation.

"I thought I was weak because I was still hurting two months in," says Lena, a shoulder surgery patient. "Turns out, my nerve was compressed. I needed more than just Tylenol—I needed answers."

Can't Bend? Can't Snap? Can't Stop Laughing!

Jason M. Aucoin

Understanding the timeline of pain helps prevent unnecessary panic—and makes sure you know when to ask for help.

Pain Scales and Communication with Healthcare Providers

You'll be asked this a lot: "What's your pain level on a scale from 0 to 10?"

It's not a trick question. It's a tool. But if you're someone who doesn't like to "complain," you might underreport.

Pro tip: Be honest. Your care team can't help you manage what they don't know exists. Use real-life analogies:
- "It feels like stabbing when I walk."
- "It's a burning sensation, especially at night."
- "I can't sleep more than two hours at a time."

Pain isn't just a number—it's a story. Tell yours clearly.

Medication Management

Opioid Use, Risks, and Tapering

Opioids can be lifesavers for post-op pain—but they come with baggage: constipation, fogginess, dependency risk.

Doctors usually prescribe them for short-term use only—3 to 10 days in many cases. After that, tapering off slowly can help avoid withdrawal symptoms.

Tips for tapering:
- Take only as needed, not "just in case."
- Switch to over-the-counter (OTC) meds early when possible.
- Talk to your doctor before stopping cold turkey.

"I kept a notebook to track when I took meds," said Darren, a hip replacement patient. *"It helped me see that I was relying less on them by week two."*

Non-Opioid Alternatives

These include:
- NSAIDs (like ibuprofen or celecoxib) to reduce inflammation
- Acetaminophen for general pain relief
- Topicals (gels, patches, creams)
- Nerve medications (gabapentin, pregabalin) for nerve-related pain

Packing Tips, Mental Prep, and All the Weird Stuff Nobody Told You About

These are often used in combination with opioids early on to lower total dosage needs.

Managing Side Effects of Pain Medications

Let's talk side effects. These can be annoying at best and dangerous at worst:
- Constipation: Use stool softeners from day one.
- Nausea: Ask for anti-nausea meds if needed.
- Drowsiness: Don't drive or make big decisions.
- Mood swings: Common with both opioids and withdrawal. Let someone know if you feel off.

Non-Pharmacological Pain Control Strategies

Let's be real—pills alone won't cut it. These strategies are not just "nice to have," they're powerful pain management tools.

Cryotherapy and Heat Therapy
- Cold (cryotherapy) helps with swelling and early inflammation.
- Use an ice machine or gel packs.
- Limit to 20-minute sessions, multiple times per day.

"I called my ice machine my new best friend," joked Mel, who had ACL reconstruction. "It's the only thing that made the throbbing manageable."

- Heat therapy helps later in recovery to relax muscles, especially during stretching and rehab.

Compression Techniques
- Compression sleeves or wraps reduce swelling and increase circulation.
- They're especially helpful with knees, ankles, and elbows.
- Make sure they're not too tight—cutting off circulation won't help anyone.

Elevation and Positioning
Gravity is your ally. Keep your limb elevated above heart level to reduce swelling. And mind your sleep position—it makes a big difference:
- Use pillows to support your operated joint.
- Side-sleepers: body pillows can help keep hips and knees aligned.

Pain is not weakness—it's a signal. Learn to understand it, manage it, and talk about it. Use all the tools in the toolbox: meds, ice, elevation, breathing, patience. And remember—this phase is temporary. You're not alone, and you're not broken.

Can't Bend? Can't Snap? Can't Stop Laughing!

Jason M. Aucoin

"I thought the pain meant something was wrong," says Amanda, recovering from shoulder arthroscopy. "But I learned pain was just part of the climb back to normal. And that I was stronger than I thought."

Sleep Strategies While Managing Pain

One of the cruelest tricks of post-surgical recovery? The moment you finally lie down to rest, your joint starts screaming. Pain often spikes at night due to reduced distractions, less movement, and increased swelling from the day.

```
Tips to get real sleep while healing:
```
- Elevate the affected joint—gravity helps reduce fluid buildup.
- Use pillows to create a "nest"—support under the knees, behind the back, or between legs can offload pressure points.
- Time your meds right—take your pain medication about 30 minutes before bed, not after you're already uncomfortable.
- Cool the joint down—ice for 20 minutes before bed can dull nerve pain and reduce inflammation.
- Try calming routines: Warm baths, white noise, and even lavender aromatherapy can help tell your brain it's bedtime, not pain time.

"I slept in a recliner for two weeks after my shoulder surgery," says Paul, 54. "It wasn't glamorous, but it was the only way I could actually sleep through the night."

Breakthrough Pain: When and How to Address It

Even with a good routine, pain can sneak up like an unexpected bill. That's breakthrough pain—those sharp spikes that break through your usual management plan.

This doesn't mean you're doing something wrong. It just means your pain needs a bit more support at that moment.

What to do:
- Identify a trigger: Did you walk more today? Skip a dose? Sleep awkwardly?
- Use your as-needed meds appropriately—don't "tough it out" to the point of misery.
- Track patterns—a pain journal (paper or app-based) can help spot trends or escalating issues.

When to worry:

Packing Tips, Mental Prep, and All the Weird Stuff Nobody Told You About

- If breakthrough pain becomes frequent or stops responding to your usual relief methods, talk to your provider. It could signal a complication or need for a plan revision.

Transitioning Off Pain Medications

There comes a point in every recovery where you ask: Do I still need this pill?

Tapering off pain meds, especially opioids, should be gradual and intentional.

Tapering tips:
- Cut your dose slowly: from two pills to one, then half, then none.
- Replace with OTC meds as advised.
- Use non-drug pain strategies (cold, stretching, and massage) more frequently.
- Don't rush if you're not ready—but don't wait until dependency sets in either.

"I was scared of the pain coming back if I stopped," says Jenna, post-hip replacement. "But I found that by week three, I wasn't even reaching for my meds anymore. I just needed the confidence to try."

Chronic Post-Surgical Pain: When to Seek Help

If you're three, four, even six months out from surgery and still in significant pain, don't just chalk it up to "normal."

Possible causes of chronic post-surgical pain include:
- Nerve damage or irritation
- Scar tissue adhesions
- Implant misalignment
- Undiagnosed complications like infection or joint instability

Signs it's time to see a specialist:
- Pain that worsens over time instead of improving
- Persistent numbness, tingling, or burning
- Pain limiting your ability to function despite therapy

Ask your doctor about a referral to a:
- Pain specialist
- Orthopedic surgeon
- Neurologist or physical medicine expert

Pain Management for Different Activity Levels

Can't Bend? Can't Snap? Can't Stop Laughing!

Jason M. Aucoin

Your body will talk to you during recovery—especially when you start moving again. But pain shouldn't be the narrator.

Here's how pain and activity relate:

- Light activity (short walks, gentle range-of-motion): mild soreness is OK; sharp pain is not.
- Moderate activity (stairs, light resistance training): expect some muscle fatigue, but joint pain should be temporary.
- High activity (returning to sports, impact movements): only attempt when cleared by your provider and after building a strong base through therapy.

Listen for warning signs:
- Pain that lingers past 24–48 hours after activity
- Pain that interrupts sleep
- Swelling, clicking, or instability in the joint

Use these to adjust:
- Rest and ice days
- Compression wraps post-activity
- Reduced loads or repetitions

"Every time I tried to push harder, my body pushed back," says Tim, an avid runner post-knee surgery. "Once I learned to progress smarter, not faster, the pain actually backed off."

Pain after joint surgery isn't a villain—it's your body's way of healing. But you don't have to suffer silently. Mix the right medications, mental strategies, physical tools, and professional support to keep pain in its place—as a phase, not a prison.

Packing Tips, Mental Prep, and All the Weird Stuff Nobody Told You About

19

Physical Therapy: Love it or Hate it, You Need It

For many, the hardest part of joint surgery isn't the surgery—it's what comes after: the sweaty, slow, sometimes tearful journey of physical therapy. Whether you enter it with hope or dread, physical therapy (PT) is the bridge between having the surgery and living your life again.

Some patients fall in love with it. Others? They fantasize about setting their resistance bands on fire. But no matter where you fall on the PT affection spectrum, one truth holds:

You cannot recover well without it.

The Science behind Rehabilitation

How PT Promotes Healing and Recovery

Here's the short story: PT tells your body what to do with the healing power it naturally has. Without movement and guided strengthening, joints stiffen, muscles shrink, and your brain forgets how to use your limb the way it used to.

PT helps by:
- Stimulating blood flow, which brings oxygen and nutrients to surgical sites.
- Strengthening surrounding muscles to protect the healing joint.
- Retraining the brain and nervous system to restore balance, control, and coordination.
- Breaking up scar tissue, which can otherwise limit motion permanently.

Jason M. Aucoin

Even passive range-of-motion exercises early on can prevent major setbacks like joint contracture or frozen limbs.

"PT saved me," says Naomi, 63, after rotator cuff surgery. *"I almost gave up until I realized each grimace was progress in disguise."*

Setting Realistic Expectations and Goals

Most patients want to recover fast—but not everyone knows what "normal" recovery looks like.

- A total knee replacement patient might need 3–6 months of PT.
- A rotator cuff repair? Closer to 6–9 months for full return to activity.
- Minor arthroscopy? Sometimes 2–6 weeks is enough.

Setting SMART goals (Specific, Measurable, Achievable, Relevant, Time-bound) with your PT can help keep motivation high even when progress feels slow.

Remember: Your progress is yours—don't compare your pace to anyone else's.

Finding the Right Physical Therapist

Your orthopedic surgeon might refer you to a clinic, but that doesn't mean it's your only option. Not all PTs are created equal, and the right therapist can make a huge difference in your experience.

Specialty Certifications to Look For

Look for credentials that match your condition:

- OCS (Orthopedic Clinical Specialist) – trained in treating musculoskeletal conditions.
- SCS (Sports Clinical Specialist) – great for athletic recovery or return-to-sport goals.
- Cert. MDT – skilled in McKenzie Method, used in back and spine rehab.
- Manual therapy certifications – for hands-on techniques in joint mobilization.

Bonus points if they've treated a lot of cases like yours.

"I switched therapists after the first one rushed me through exercises," says Kevin, who had ACL reconstruction. *"The second one specialized in sports knees. Night and day difference."*

Questions to Ask Before Starting

- How many patients like me have you treated?

Packing Tips, Mental Prep, and All the Weird Stuff Nobody Told You About

- What's your typical approach for [insert your surgery]?
- Will I work with the same therapist every session?
- How do you track progress?
- Can I contact you between sessions?

Don't be afraid to treat your first visit like a job interview—you're hiring someone to rebuild your body.

Your First PT Session: What to Expect

So, what happens when you walk—or hobble—into your first session?

Here's a breakdown:
- Initial Assessment: They'll measure your range of motion, strength, balance, and pain levels. Expect questions about pain location, mobility challenges, and daily function.
- Goal Setting: Your therapist will collaborate with you to define short- and long-term recovery goals.
- Education: Expect a walkthrough of your anatomy, healing timeline, and what to expect in future sessions.
- Light Activity: You might do basic exercises like heel slides, quad sets, ankle pumps, or assisted stretches. It won't be a boot camp...yet.
- Homework: You'll be given a home exercise program (HEP)—and yes, you're expected to actually do it.

Pro tip: Keep a notebook or app log of your exercises and symptoms. It helps track progress and identify issues early.

"After my first shoulder PT, I was sore, tired, and weirdly proud," says Julia, 44. "It was the first time I felt like I was doing something to heal, not just waiting."
Let's continue Chapter 20 with the next sections, keeping our engaging, informative style rooted in relatable insights and real-world voices.

Home Exercise Programs: Making Them Work

Your physical therapist may only see you two or three times a week, but you live with your body every day. That's why the Home Exercise Program (HEP) is just as important—sometimes more so—than what happens in the clinic.

Creating a Sustainable Routine

Can't Bend? Can't Snap? Can't Stop Laughing!

Jason M. Aucoin

A good HEP is like brushing your teeth: simple, consistent, and daily. But unlike brushing your teeth, it may make you sweat and swear.

Here's how to make it doable:
- Schedule it like any other appointment. Pick a regular time.
- Break it up if you need to—morning stretches, evening strength.
- Use cues like TV time or meal prep as reminders to do your exercises.
- Pair it with habit triggers (like coffee or music) to make it more enjoyable.

"I did my knee exercises during commercial breaks," says Maria, a 70-year-old knee replacement patient. *"Now my grandkids call it my 'Netflix PT.' it stuck."*

Consistency matters more than intensity. Think marathon, not sprint.

Tracking Progress Effectively

Progress in rehab is rarely a straight line. One week you'll feel like a rock star, the next week you'll wonder if you're going backwards.

Track these metrics:
- Range of motion (can you bend more today than last week?)
- Strength (can you do more reps or hold positions longer?)
- Pain scale (is discomfort decreasing over time?)
- Function (can you do more daily tasks with less effort?)

Use a journal, a rehab app, or even your phone's Notes app to jot down changes. When you're discouraged, looking back can reveal how far you've really come.

When PT Hurts: Distinguishing Good Pain from Bad

Let's clear this up: rehab pain is normal—but not all pain is good.

Good pain = muscle soreness, stretch discomfort, effort-based fatigue.
Bad pain = sharp, stabbing, burning, or swelling that worsens after rest.

Red flags:
- Pain that wakes you up at night.
- Pain that lingers hours after exercise.
- Sudden loss of range of motion or function.

"I kept pushing because I thought I had to," says Jake, a former college soccer player recovering from ACL surgery. *"Turned out I was tearing at scar tissue that wasn't ready. I lost two weeks of progress."*

Communicate with your PT. They can adjust reps, modify positions, or refer you back to your surgeon if something's off.

Packing Tips, Mental Prep, and All the Weird Stuff Nobody Told You About

Plateaus and Breakthroughs in Rehabilitation

Every rehab journey hits the dreaded plateau. You're showing up, doing the work... and seeing no gains. It's demoralizing, and it's common.

Here's why it happens:
- Healing slows as tissue matures.
- You've reached the point where gains require more nuanced movement.
- The nervous system needs time to rewire itself.

Here's what helps:
- Change up your routine. New exercises can challenge muscles differently.
- Celebrate small wins—stairs without pain, a deeper bend, a quicker walk.
- Focus on function, not just numbers. Can you drive? Get off the floor? Return to work?

"I was stuck at 90 degrees of knee bend for two weeks," says Delilah. *"Then one day—bam—97. I cried in the clinic. That little bend felt like Everest."*

Trust the process. Plateaus often come right before breakthroughs.

PT for Different Personality Types

Physical therapy isn't one-size-fits-all. How you approach it can make or break your progress.

For the Overachiever: Avoiding Setbacks

You know who you are. You're the patient trying to jump stairs three weeks post-op or sneak into spin class at week four. You see PT as a race, and you want to win.

But here's the thing: tissue healing has a biological timeline. You can't rush collagen.

Overdoing it can lead to:
- Inflammation
- Re-tears or setbacks
- Longer overall recovery

Tips:
- Channel that energy into perfect form, not heavier reps.
- Ask your PT how to measure smart progress.

Can't Bend? Can't Snap? Can't Stop Laughing!

- Accept that rest is productive, too.

"I tore my meniscus redo because I tried to 'crush' rehab," admits Ron, a former marathoner. *"The second time, I learned to respect the process."*

For the Reluctant: Finding Motivation

Maybe you hate exercise. Maybe it hurts. Maybe you're overwhelmed.

Whatever the reason, you're not lazy—you're human. But without regular PT, you risk:
- Poor long-term function
- Increased pain and stiffness
- Permanent loss of motion

Motivational hacks:
- Break exercises into 5-minute chunks.
- Make a recovery playlist or watch a favorite show during sessions.
- Track your progress visually—seeing gains is empowering.
- Pair up with a rehab buddy, even virtually.

"I dreaded therapy," says Shirley, who had shoulder surgery at 68. *"My daughter started texting me daily reminders—and then joined me for stretching. It turned into bonding."*

PT doesn't have to be perfect. It just has to be **consistent**.

Alternative Therapies to Complement PT

Sometimes, healing calls for more than just mat exercises and resistance bands. Complementary therapies can fill in the gaps, reduce pain, and restore confidence—especially during tough rehab days.

Aquatic Therapy

Water has a magical quality when it comes to joint rehab. The buoyancy unloads joints, while the resistance builds strength.

Benefits:
- Reduces weight-bearing stress
- Improves range of motion safely
- Builds strength without strain

It's especially helpful for:
- Post-op knee and hip patients
- Patients with arthritis or weight-related challenges

Packing Tips, Mental Prep, and All the Weird Stuff Nobody Told You About

- Anyone struggling with pain during land-based therapy

"I was scared to bend my knee after surgery," says Phillip, a 64-year-old total knee patient. "In the pool, I could move freely. I felt like I had my body back."

Many rehab centers and YMCAs offer warm-water pools for therapeutic use—worth checking out if you're feeling stuck or sore.

Manual Therapy Approaches

Sometimes, the hands of a skilled therapist make all the difference.

Manual therapy may include:
- Soft tissue mobilization
- Joint mobilization
- Myofascial release
- Trigger point therapy

These techniques aim to reduce scar tissue buildup, improve joint glide, and ease muscular tightness that limits movement.

"After shoulder surgery, my arm felt glued to my side," says Grace, a 45-year-old desk worker. "Manual therapy loosened up the tight spots I didn't even know were there."

Pro tip: Not all PTs specialize in hands-on work, so ask if they offer it—or if they can refer you to someone who does.

Transitioning from Formal PT to Lifelong Maintenance

At some point, your regular PT visits will end—but your rehab doesn't.

Graduation day isn't the finish line. It's a pivot point from guided therapy to self-guided maintenance.

Tips for transitioning:
- Get a written home program tailored to your progress.
- Ask for guidance on gym equipment or community classes.
- Schedule a "tune-up" PT session every few months if needed.
- Set personal goals—like hiking again, lifting grandkids, or returning to sports.

"My PT gave me a post-discharge 'menu' of exercises," says Josh, a 39-year-old hip labral repair patient. "Now I rotate them each week like a workout plan."

Can't Bend? Can't Snap? Can't Stop Laughing!

Jason M. Aucoin

Rehab may end, but body care doesn't. The goal is lifelong function, not just short-term recovery.

Insurance Coverage and Advocating for Needed Sessions

One of the biggest frustrations? Hitting your insurance limit before you hit your goals.

Here's the reality:
- Many plans cap therapy sessions at 20–30 per year.
- Some require pre-authorizations, others cut off when "progress" slows.

Here's what you can do:
- Appeal if you're denied sessions—your PT can write a letter of medical necessity.
- Ask your provider for cash-pay options, which can be surprisingly affordable.
- Consider group rehab classes, which are often cheaper and still effective.
- Use Flexible Spending Accounts (FSA) or Health Savings Accounts (HSA) for coverage.

"I hit my limit at 14 sessions," says Natalie, a teacher recovering from rotator cuff repair. "My PT helped me design a hybrid program—two in-person visits a month and home check-ins. It saved me."

Also, advocate early—before you're cut off. Let your PT know your financial and insurance boundaries upfront so you can work together on a realistic plan.

PT Is a Partnership

Whether you're Type A or Type "I'll do it tomorrow," physical therapy thrives on collaboration. The best outcomes don't come from heroic bursts of effort, but from steady, tailored work over time—with a therapist who sees the whole you.

"Rehab changed me," says Stephanie, a 62-year-old double hip replacement survivor. "It taught me to move again—but also to trust my body, be patient, and take ownership."

So love it or hate it, physical therapy is your ally. Show up. Do the work. Keep the long game in sight.

Packing Tips, Mental Prep, and All the Weird Stuff Nobody Told You About

20 Complications to Watch For

No one goes into surgery dreaming about complications. Still, it's crucial to know what's normal, what's not, and what to do if the road to recovery throws you a curveball. Being informed doesn't mean being anxious—it means being prepared.

Normal vs. Abnormal Post-Operative Symptoms

After joint surgery, discomfort is expected. So is swelling. And stiffness. But where's the line between normal healing and a red flag?

What's Normal (in the first few days to weeks):
- Swelling that improves when elevated
- Bruising near the surgical site
- Incisional soreness
- General fatigue
- Mild stiffness that gradually improves

What's Not Normal?
- Redness spreading beyond the incision
- Fever over 101°F (38.3°C)
- Drainage that's yellow, green, or foul-smelling
- Intense pain that worsens instead of improving
- Sudden swelling in one leg, especially with warmth or discoloration

"I didn't realize my low-grade fever was a sign of infection until it spiked," recalls Diane, a 58-year-old shoulder surgery patient. "Thank goodness I called when I did."

Can't Bend? Can't Snap? Can't Stop Laughing!

Jason M. Aucoin

The bottom line: If something feels off, don't wait. Reach out.

Infection: Prevention, Signs, and Management

Infections can range from mild nuisances to serious complications requiring re-operation. But the good news? They're often preventable.

Wound Care Best Practices

Cleanliness isn't optional. It's essential.

Basic wound care rules:
- Keep the incision dry for the first few days or as instructed
- Always wash your hands before touching the area
- Change dressings only as advised—more isn't better
- Avoid soaking in baths, pools, or hot tubs until fully cleared

"I thought my incision looked dry, so I stopped covering it. A week later, it started oozing," shares Reggie, a 42-year-old ACL reconstruction patient. *"I didn't realize early exposure was risky."*

Follow your discharge instructions to the letter. They're there to protect you.

When to Call Your Surgeon Immediately

Call your surgeon or provider right away if you experience:
- Increased redness or warmth around the incision
- Pus-like drainage
- A fever over 101°F (38.3°C)
- Chills or flu-like symptoms
- A foul smell from the incision
- Sudden sharp pain at the surgical site

Don't hesitate or try to "wait it out." Early intervention can save your joint—and your peace of mind.

Blood Clots: Risk Factors and Prevention

Blood clots, particularly deep vein thrombosis (DVT) and pulmonary embolism (PE), are serious risks after joint surgery—especially in the lower limbs. But awareness and action can keep you safe.

DVT and PE Warning Signs

Packing Tips, Mental Prep, and All the Weird Stuff Nobody Told You About

DVT (Deep Vein Thrombosis) usually shows up in the leg:
- Swelling (especially on one side)
- Warmth to the touch
- Red or purplish skin discoloration
- Cramping pain, often in the calf or thigh

PE (Pulmonary Embolism) happens when a clot travels to the lungs:
- Sudden shortness of breath
- Chest pain, especially when breathing deeply
- Rapid heart rate
- Coughing (sometimes with blood)

"I thought I was just winded from moving around," says Lena, a 70-year-old hip replacement patient. "But when my heart started racing, I knew something was wrong."

These aren't "wait and see" symptoms—call emergency services immediately.

Anticoagulation Management

To prevent clots, your provider may prescribe:
- Blood thinners (like warfarin, rivaroxaban, or heparin)
- Compression stockings
- Intermittent pneumatic compression devices
- Early mobility protocols (walking, ankle pumps, leg lifts)

Take medications exactly as directed. Missing doses—or stopping too early—can be dangerous.

Always alert your care team if:
- You experience unusual bruising
- You have a history of bleeding disorders
- You're on other meds that may interact

And most importantly, get moving (safely and slowly). Sitting still is the enemy of circulation.

Nerve Damage: Temporary vs. Permanent

Nerves are delicate messengers. Sometimes, during surgery—even with precision—they can get jostled, stretched, or nicked. Most of the time, it's temporary. Occasionally, it's not.

Can't Bend? Can't Snap? Can't Stop Laughing!

Jason M. Aucoin

Paresthesia, Numbness, and Weakness

You might wake up from surgery and feel like your skin's asleep—or discover a patch of numbness near the incision or down a limb. This tingling, known as paresthesia, often resolves in weeks or months.

"After my shoulder surgery, I couldn't feel my pinky for three months," recalls Pete, a 38-year-old rock climber. "It was freaky at first, but my doc reassured me it wasn't permanent."

But not all nerve damage is benign. Signs of more serious nerve involvement include:
- Persistent muscle weakness
- Complete loss of sensation in an area
- Electric shock-like pain or burning
- No improvement over 6–12 weeks

Always report these symptoms. Nerve conduction studies or EMGs might be recommended to assess the extent of injury.

Recovery Timeframes and Expectations

Nerve tissue heals slowly. The common saying is 1 millimeter per day, or roughly 1 inch per month, depending on the type and location of the nerve.

Here's what you might expect:
- Minor bruising/stretching: Recovery in weeks to a few months
- More serious but incomplete damage: 6–12 months or longer
- Severed or permanently injured nerves: May not fully recover, but options like nerve grafts, physical therapy, or pain management can help

Keep hope: even slow progress is still progress. Many patients regain full function with time and support.

Hardware Issues and Implant Complications

Joint implants, screws, plates—they're marvels of modern medicine. But just like any tech, things can occasionally go sideways.

Loosening, Dislocation, and Failure

Implants don't last forever. Some patients never have problems. Others? Complications can arise.

Signs your implant might be acting up:

Packing Tips, Mental Prep, and All the Weird Stuff Nobody Told You About

- A sudden pop or shift in joint alignment
- Increased pain or grinding sensations
- A feeling of instability or "giving way"
- Decreased range of motion after initial improvements

Common issues include:
- Loosening: The bond between bone and implant weakens over time or due to improper healing
- Dislocation: More common in hip or shoulder replacements—where ball-and-socket movement can slip
- Fracture: Around or near the implant, often from trauma or bone weakness
- Mechanical wear: Especially in older or high-activity patients

"I was feeling great until I stepped sideways and felt my hip shift," says Claire, who later learned her implant had slightly dislocated. *"I thought I was back to square one—but I wasn't. It was fixable."*

Allergic Reactions to Materials

Rare but real: some patients react to metals used in implants (like nickel, cobalt, or chromium).

Symptoms may include:
- Rash or skin irritation near the implant
- Persistent swelling without infection
- Joint pain without an obvious cause

If you have a known metal allergy—or develop unexplained symptoms—your provider may order testing or imaging. In severe cases, implant replacement might be considered using hypoallergenic alternatives like ceramic or titanium.

Stiffness and Range of Motion Concerns

The fear is real: "What if I never move like I used to?"

Stiffness after joint surgery is incredibly common—especially if you delay movement, avoid PT, or experience excessive scar tissue buildup.

Adhesive Capsulitis Prevention

Also known as frozen joint syndrome, adhesive capsulitis happens when the soft tissue around the joint becomes inflamed and tight, limiting mobility.

Common risk factors:

Can't Bend? Can't Snap? Can't Stop Laughing!

- Inactivity post-surgery
- Diabetes or thyroid disorders
- Poor pain control (which can reduce willingness to move)

Prevention strategies:
- Start PT as soon as your surgeon gives the green light
- Don't skip home exercises (even when it's hard or boring)
- Communicate if pain is stopping you from moving—adjustments can be made
- Use gentle mobility aids (like continuous passive motion machines for the knee)

"I skipped PT for two weeks after my rotator cuff repair, and boom—frozen shoulder," says Ana, 51. "It added four extra months of rehab. I'll never do that again."

Mild stiffness usually resolves with consistent effort. Severe cases might require manipulation under anesthesia (MUA) or even revision surgery—but these are typically last resorts.

Breaking Through Motion Restrictions

So, you're doing the stretches. You're going to PT. And yet... your joint still feels like it's moving through molasses. This is one of the most frustrating parts of recovery: plateauing in range of motion.

Why it happens:
- Scar tissue buildup
- Joint capsule stiffness
- Guarded movement due to pain or fear
- Inadequate physical therapy intensity or frequency

What can help:
- Manual therapy: A skilled PT using hands-on techniques to mobilize tissue
- Instrument-assisted soft tissue mobilization (IASTM): Think "muscle scraping" to break adhesions
- Prolonged stretching sessions: Holding positions for 2–5 minutes
- Modalities like heat therapy before movement to loosen tight areas
- Hydrotherapy: Warm water exercises reduce resistance and pain
- Home splinting: Devices that gently and passively push joints toward better mobility

"My surgeon said I might never fully bend my knee again," says Tariq, who had a total knee replacement. "But with aggressive PT, a ton of tears, and six months of stretching—I hit 120 degrees."

Success takes persistence. Celebrate small improvements. A few degrees more today can mean walking pain-free tomorrow.

Packing Tips, Mental Prep, and All the Weird Stuff Nobody Told You About

Delayed and Non-Union Issues

Bone healing is a beautiful thing... until it's not.

A delayed union means the bone is healing, just more slowly than expected. A non-union means the bone isn't healing on its own at all.

Signs include:
- Persistent pain at the fracture or surgical site
- No improvement on X-rays over months
- Swelling or instability when bearing weight

Causes:
- Smoking (biggest culprit)
- Poor nutrition or Vitamin D deficiency
- Certain meds like NSAIDs or steroids
- Infections
- Poor fixation (hardware doesn't support the bone well)

What can be done:
- Bone stimulators: Ultrasound or electrical devices to encourage bone growth
- Grafting: Adding bone tissue (from the patient or a donor) to restart healing
- Revision surgery: Replacing or reinforcing failed hardware

Healing bones need the right biological environment—give yours the best shot with good nutrition, no nicotine, and regular follow-ups.

Prosthetic Joint Infection

Here's the tough truth: even years after joint replacement, infection can still strike.

How? Bacteria from dental work, UTIs, or skin wounds can enter the bloodstream and settle around a prosthetic joint.

Warning signs include:
- Sudden joint pain after being pain-free
- Swelling, redness, or warmth around the joint
- Drainage from the surgical site—even long after healing
- Fever, chills, or fatigue without another clear source

Prevention tips:
- Take antibiotics before certain dental or surgical procedures if recommended
- Treat infections elsewhere in the body quickly
- Keep the area around the joint clean and moisturized (but not overly moist)

Can't Bend? Can't Snap? Can't Stop Laughing!

If infection is suspected, you may need:
- Blood tests and joint fluid aspiration
- Antibiotics via IV or oral route
- In some cases, removal and replacement of the prosthesis

"Ten years after my hip replacement, I got a weird fever," recalls Lisa. *"Turned out to be an infection in the implant. Luckily, we caught it early, and antibiotics saved me from another surgery."*

Creating Your Personal Warning Signs Checklist

Everyone's risk factors are different, which means your red flag list should be customized.

What to include:
- Your surgery type and known complication risks
- Current medications (especially blood thinners, immunosuppressants)
- Known allergies (including to implants or medications)
- Medical history (like diabetes, clotting disorders, previous infections)
- Surgeon or hospital contact info

Sample Checklist:
- ☐ Sudden or worsening joint pain after progress
- ☐ Redness, heat, or pus at incision
- ☐ New fever over 100.4°F (38°C)
- ☐ Leg swelling or calf pain
- ☐ Chest pain or shortness of breath
- ☐ Numbness or tingling not improving
- ☐ Audible pop or joint instability

Print this out, stick it on your fridge, and share with your caregiver or loved one.

Building Your Medical Emergency Plan

In post-op life, preparedness is power. Emergencies can happen fast, especially in the first 3 months. Here's how to stay ready:

```
1. Know your nearest ER
```
- Which hospitals are in-network?
- Does your surgeon have admitting privileges there?

```
2. Keep your med and surgery summary on hand
```
- Surgery date
- Type of procedure
- Implants used

Packing Tips, Mental Prep, and All the Weird Stuff Nobody Told You About

- Allergies and current meds

3. Create a care circle
- One or two trusted people who know your recovery plan
- Make sure they have your checklist and surgeon's info

4. Pack a "go bag" (just in case)

ID and insurance cards

Med list and pill bottles

Comfortable clothes

A copy of your discharge and implant papers

5. Use tech wisely

Set reminders for meds and symptoms to watch

Use apps like MyChart for fast communication with your surgeon's office

"I had chest pain three days after surgery and didn't want to 'overreact,'" says Jamal. "I'm glad I called. I had a small PE—and the ER doc said quick action saved me."

Can't Bend? Can't Snap? Can't Stop Laughing!

Jason M. Aucoin

21
Tools and Gadgets That Help you Heal Smarter

Cold Therapy Systems

Post-op swelling and pain don't stand a chance when you've got the right cooling gear. But not all ice packs are created equal.

Comparing Ice Machines and Wraps

Ice Machines (a.k.a. Cold Therapy Units):
These circulate ice water through a wrap using a small pump. Brands like CryoCuff, Polar Care, and Game Ready are popular.

Pros:
- Consistent cooling
- Less mess and melting
- Hands-free application
- Some combine compression for added relief

Cons:
- More expensive (anywhere from $100–$400+)
- Needs power (or batteries)
- Not always covered by insurance

Reusable Gel Wraps:
Simple, effective, and budget-friendly. Brands like TheraPearl or Chattanooga work well when chilled properly.

Pros:

- Affordable
- Flexible for different joints
- No wires or batteries

Cons:
- Needs frequent re-cooling
- Can warm up quickly
- Not as effective for large swelling

DIY vs. Commercial Solutions

DIY Options:
- Bag of frozen peas (classic, but leaky)
- Ziplock bag with water + rubbing alcohol = super moldable
- Towel-wrapped ice packs

These work in a pinch, but for major surgeries, many patients say the commercial cold therapy units are game-changers.

"I didn't think I needed the ice machine until I went one night without it. Never again," says Troy, after ACL reconstruction.

Mobility Aids and When to Use Them

Mobility aids are not signs of weakness—they're keys to safe movement. The trick is knowing which one to use and when.

Crutches, Canes, and Walkers

- Crutches: Standard post-op gear. Great for non-weight-bearing periods, but take coordination.
- Forearm crutches: More ergonomic for longer-term use.
- Canes: Best for minor balance issues or light support during later recovery stages.
- Walkers: Offer more stability, especially for elderly patients or those recovering from hip/knee replacements.

Pro tip: Don't wait until you fall to ask for a walker. If your PT or surgeon suggests one, it's for a good reason.

Knee Scooters and Wheelchairs

Can't Bend? Can't Snap? Can't Stop Laughing!

Jason M. Aucoin

- Knee Scooters: Fantastic for foot/ankle surgeries. You can roll around without hopping or tiring yourself out.
  - Watch for obstacles and rug edges
  - Consider outdoor vs. indoor use
- Wheelchairs: Used less often in elective ortho surgeries but essential after complex or multi-joint procedures.

"The knee scooter saved my sanity," laughs Marsha, post-bunion surgery. *"I could cook dinner again—even if it was just boxed mac & cheese."*

Bathroom Safety Equipment

Let's be honest: the bathroom becomes an obstacle course after surgery. These gadgets help make it safer and way less stressful.

Shower Chairs and Transfer Benches

- Shower Chair: Allows you to sit while washing up—especially important if you're woozy or can't bear weight.
- Transfer Bench: Extends beyond the tub edge so you can sit down outside the tub and scoot in safely.

Bonus Tip: Use a handheld showerhead to avoid awkward twisting. Suction cup grab bars are not reliable—install fixed ones when possible.

Raised Toilet Seats and Grab Bars

After hip or knee surgery, sitting low can be painful—or risky.

- Raised Toilet Seat: Adds height so you don't strain. Some models attach to your existing toilet; others come as standalone commodes.
- Grab Bars: Help with standing and balance. Install them beside the toilet and shower.

"It's not glamorous, but my raised seat was my favorite purchase post-op," says Dean, recovering from hip replacement.

Dressing and Grooming Aids

Putting on socks shouldn't feel like a triathlon. These tools make daily routines doable again—especially when bending, twisting, or balancing is a no-go.

Packing Tips, Mental Prep, and All the Weird Stuff Nobody Told You About

Reachers and Grabbers

These long-handled tools are your new best friends.

- Pick up dropped items
- Pull clothing over your feet
- Open curtains, retrieve light laundry, grab snacks from high shelves (no shame)

Look for a grabber with a rubberized grip and a rotating head for added functionality. You'll be surprised how often you use it—even after you're better.

Sock Aids and Dressing Sticks

- Sock Aid: This foam-lined plastic sleeve lets you slide your foot into a sock without bending over. It feels weird the first time, but it works like magic.
- Dressing Stick: Great for maneuvering shirts, jackets, or pants over your limbs. Also helps push or pull clothing into place.

Bonus grooming tips:
- Long-handled sponges or loofahs are great for showering.
- Electric razors reduce the need for awkward arm positions.
- Dry shampoo and face/body wipes are gold when full showers are hard.

"I used to laugh at the sock aid on hospital supply lists. Then I needed it every morning. Total lifesaver," says Brian, post-spine surgery.

Kitchen Modifications and Tools

Cooking post-surgery is tricky unless your kitchen does some of the work for you.

- High stools or rolling chairs for meal prep without standing
- Non-slip cutting boards and adaptive knives (like rocker knives)
- Electric can openers and jar grips
- One-handed prep tools if one arm or hand is out of commission

Keep essentials on the counter or in an accessible cart—no need to reach or stoop.

Meal hacks:
- Prep freezer meals before surgery
- Use a slow cooker, rice cooker, or air fryer (push-button meals!)
- Silicone grips or easy-pour kettles help avoid spills and burns

Bedroom Setup for Recovery

Can't Bend? Can't Snap? Can't Stop Laughing!

Jason M. Aucoin

The bedroom becomes command central during recovery. Make it ergonomic and recovery-friendly.

Bed Positioning Systems

- Bed wedges help elevate legs or back without stacking pillows (they never stay put).
- Adjustable beds (if you have one) are a dream post-op.
- Over-bed tables let you eat, read, or work from bed comfortably.

Pro tip: Keep meds, water, tissues, and your phone charger within arm's reach. A small nightstand caddy or bed rail organizer is perfect.

Transfer Aids

- Bed rails: Assist with getting in and out of bed safely.
- Leg lifters: Long straps that help lift heavy or weak legs into bed.
- Slide sheets or transfer boards: Useful if you need assistance from a caregiver or are recovering from multi-joint surgery.

Pain Management Devices

Technology that helps you hurt less without drugs? Sign us up.

TENS Units

Transcutaneous Electrical Nerve Stimulation (TENS) uses low-voltage electrical pulses to interrupt pain signals.

When it works:
- After soft tissue surgery or during chronic flare-ups
- With guidance from your PT or doctor

Pros:
- Non-invasive
- Can use several times a day
- Compact and portable

Watch-outs:
Avoid if you have a pacemaker or certain implants.

Massage Tools

Packing Tips, Mental Prep, and All the Weird Stuff Nobody Told You About

- Percussion massagers like Theragun or Hypervolt can help with stiffness and scar tissue—but use cautiously after surgery.
- Foam rollers and massage balls are great for long-term recovery and maintenance.
- Heated massagers or shiatsu pads for neck, back, or shoulders—especially helpful when you're stuck in bed or the recliner.

"I swear by my TENS unit. It gave me more control over my pain—especially when I wanted to wean off meds," says Erika, rotator cuff repair patient.

Specialized Clothing and Adaptive Wear

Forget buttons and tight jeans—post-op fashion is all about function.

- Post-surgical shirts with shoulder snaps or front zippers = must-haves after shoulder, chest, or arm surgery.
- Velcro or magnetic closures instead of buttons/zippers for one-handed dressing.
- Elastic waistbands, loose-fitting joggers, or tearaway pants work wonders for hip, knee, or ankle surgery.
- Open-toe orthopedic shoes or slippers help with swelling and bandages.

Bonus: Some brands offer stylish adaptive wear that doesn't scream "hospital chic."

Technology Helpers (Apps, Smart Home Devices)

Smart tech can literally lighten your load during recovery.

- Medication tracking apps (like Medisafe) to stay on top of dosing schedules
- PT apps with video instructions and progress tracking
- Wearables (like Apple Watch, Fitbit) to monitor heart rate, sleep, or step count during rehab
- Voice assistants (Alexa, Google Home) to set reminders, control lights, or call family when hands are busy or mobility's limited
- Smart plugs/lights to control devices from bed

"I set my smart speaker to remind me to take meds and ice my knee. It became my personal nurse," says Carlos, ACL reconstruction patient.

Worth the Investment vs. Skip It: Cost-Benefit Analysis

Worth it:
- Cold therapy machine (especially for joint replacements)
- Sock aid (you'll use it daily—zero shame)
- Grabber/reacher (long-term value)

Can't Bend? Can't Snap? Can't Stop Laughing!

- Bed wedge or leg elevation system
- Shower chair and grab bars (safety first)

Skip or DIY:
- Expensive dressing sticks (some people use wooden spoons!)
- Top-tier massage guns if you're not cleared to use one
- High-end walkers unless prescribed (many can be borrowed or rented)

Consider used or refurbished equipment—check with your surgeon's office, PT clinic, or local rehab store.

Borrowing, Renting, and Insurance Coverage for Equipment

Hot tip: You may not need to buy half this stuff.

- Borrow from friends/family who've had surgery (they're often happy to offload tools they only used for a few weeks)
- Hospital loan programs sometimes offer walkers, commodes, or ice machines
- Medical equipment rental companies deliver and pick up gear
- Check insurance or FSA/HSA plans—many cover:
  - Mobility aids
  - Cold therapy devices
  - Bedside commodes
  - Home PT equipment (if prescribed)

Pro tip: Ask your PT or surgeon to write a "medical necessity" note—it can help with insurance reimbursement.

22

Returning to Normal Life (Or Your New Normal)

Surgery might be the fix, but recovery is the real journey. Whether you're aiming to get back to your job, your workouts, or just the ability to tie your own shoes without wincing—this chapter is your blueprint.

Setting Realistic Activity Timelines

Everyone asks, "How long until I'm back to normal?" The truth: it depends.

- Knee/hip replacements? Walking unassisted might take 3–6 weeks. Full return to sports? 6–12 months.
- Rotator cuff surgery? Dressing yourself without help: 4–6 weeks. Overhead strength? 6+ months.
- Spinal fusions? Sitting/standing comfortably: 2–3 months. Lifting heavy objects: maybe never, or only under guidance.

Real Talk: Don't measure success by your neighbor's timeline. Factors like age, fitness level, type of procedure, and even mental state all influence recovery.

"I was frustrated seeing other people jogging after knee surgery while I could barely walk to the mailbox. But my surgeon reminded me—I started with worse cartilage damage. Different starting lines = different finish times."

Workplace Accommodations and Returns

For many, work is the final frontier in recovery—and a major source of anxiety.

Can't Bend? Can't Snap? Can't Stop Laughing!

Legal Rights and Disability Benefits

- FMLA (Family and Medical Leave Act): Guarantees up to 12 weeks of job-protected leave (unpaid) in the U.S.
- Short-Term Disability Insurance: Usually covers 40–70% of income during recovery.
- Long-Term Disability: Kicks in if you're still unable to work after a set time (often 3–6 months).
- ADA (Americans with Disabilities Act): Requires employers to provide reasonable accommodations if you're returning with ongoing limitations.

Tip: Your doctor or PT can help document your limitations—this makes a big difference when requesting modifications.

Ergonomic Considerations

- Desk job? Ask for:
  - Adjustable chair with lumbar support
  - Keyboard trays to reduce shoulder strain
  - Sit/stand desks (especially post-spine surgery)
- On-your-feet roles?
  - Anti-fatigue mats
  - Frequent seated breaks
  - Modified duties or lighter lifting responsibilities
- Driving requirements? Make sure you're cleared to operate a vehicle safely—reaction time and range of motion matter more than you think.

"I had a custom footrest, a rolling stool, and voice-to-text software after my ankle surgery. It looked a little ridiculous—but it saved me from re-injury," says Michaela, a retail manager. Perfect—this is where things get real and relatable. Let's dig into some of the biggest "Am I allowed to do that yet?" questions people have after joint surgery.

Driving Again: Safety and Legal Considerations

Getting back behind the wheel can feel like reclaiming your independence—but don't rush it.

Key things to consider:

- Reaction Time: Can you slam on the brakes without hesitation? This is especially crucial if your surgery was on your right leg.
- Pain Medications: If you're still on opioids or sedatives, driving is legally and medically a no-go.
- Doctor's Clearance: Most surgeons won't give you the green light until:

Packing Tips, Mental Prep, and All the Weird Stuff Nobody Told You About

- You're off narcotics
- You've regained a safe range of motion
- You can perform an emergency stop simulation (sometimes tested in PT)

Rule of thumb:
- Knee/Hip Replacement: 4–6 weeks (right side), 2–3 weeks (left side with automatic transmission)
- Shoulder Surgery: 4–6 weeks (you must be able to grip, turn the wheel, and manage shifting safely)

"I practiced in an empty parking lot before returning to regular roads—just in case I'd forgotten how weird my new knee felt under pressure," said one patient recovering from TKA.

Sexual Activity after Joint Surgery

Nobody really talks about it—but you should ask.

The honest truth:
- You can generally resume sexual activity 2–6 weeks post-op, depending on the joint involved and your position flexibility.
- Pain, stiffness, and fear of hurting yourself (or your partner) are common barriers.
- Communication is everything—both with your partner and, yes, even with your healthcare provider if you're unsure what's safe.

Pro Tips:
- Hip replacement patients: Avoid positions that involve deep hip flexion or rotation early on.
- Shoulder surgery: Limit weight-bearing through the arm; find positions that allow the arm to be supported.
- Knee issues: Pillows under the knees can reduce strain and increase comfort.

"My PT handed me a one-sheet titled 'Yes, You Can Have Sex Again,' and I nearly died laughing. But honestly—it helped," shared a 52-year-old patient post-hip replacement.

Travel Planning Post-Surgery

Adventure doesn't have to wait forever—but a little planning goes a long way.

Air Travel with Joint Replacement

Can't Bend? Can't Snap? Can't Stop Laughing!

Jason M. Aucoin

Most surgeons recommend avoiding flights for 4–6 weeks post-op due to increased risk of blood clots (DVTs).

If you do have to fly:

- Wear compression stockings
- Walk or stretch every hour
- Hydrate like crazy
- Consider blood thinners if you're high risk—your doctor may prescribe a short-term course.

TSA Reality Check:
- Your implant will set off metal detectors.
- Request a pat-down or opt for a body scanner.
- Carry a card from your surgeon noting your joint replacement—it's not required, but can ease confusion.

"Security waved me over and asked, 'Hip or knee?' I said, 'Left hip, 6 months old,' and he laughed. Turns out it's common enough that they don't even blink anymore," one patient shared.

What We Wish Every Patient Knew

As we come to the final pages, here's a collection of insight from voices you've met along the way—surgeons, physical therapists, and most importantly, patients who've walked (or wheeled) this road before you. Take this as a companion to carry forward, a north star for your recovery and your future.

From the Author:

"Recovery doesn't reward perfection—it rewards persistence. You don't have to bounce back fast. You just have to keep showing up, one honest, imperfect step at a time.

From the Orthopedic Surgeon:

"We can fix the joint. But the healing? That part is yours. Respect the process, ask questions, and don't compare your path to anyone else's. Recovery is deeply personal—and so is success."

From the Physical Therapist:

Packing Tips, Mental Prep, and All the Weird Stuff Nobody Told You About

"Some days you'll feel like you're climbing a mountain in molasses. Other days you'll surprise yourself. Track the trend, not the moment. Healing isn't linear, and progress hides in the small wins."

From a Knee Replacement Patient, 9 Months Out:

"I cried more in the first 4 weeks than I expected—but then I danced at my daughter's wedding at month five. Give yourself grace. Every tear, every setback is part of the comeback."

From a Young Athlete Post-ACL Surgery:

"I thought my identity was gone. But PT taught me I was more than the sport. I rebuilt not just my leg, but my mindset. I'm stronger now—in every sense of the word."

From a 72-Year-Old Hip Replacement Patient:

"People told me I was 'too old' for surgery. Now I hike with my granddaughter. Don't let fear—or other people—make decisions for you."

From a Caregiver:

"Don't forget to take care of yourself, too. You can't pour from an empty cup. Rest, ask for help, and celebrate their progress—because you're part of it."

One Final Note:

You are not just a patient—you are a participant in your own recovery story. There will be scars. There will be setbacks. But there will also be strength, resilience, and triumph. You've come this far. You've read this far. And that means you're ready for whatever comes next.

The joint is just the beginning. The life you build after it? That's the real story.

Can't Bend? Can't Snap? Can't Stop Laughing!

Jason M. Aucoin

About the Author

Jason M. Aucoin is a medical writer, health journalist, and relentless asker of "Wait, but what actually happens next?" With a background in science communication and a knack for translating clinical jargon into everyday language, Jason has spent over a decade helping patients understand what's really going on inside their bodies—and what to expect when things go under the knife.

His work has appeared in health publications, surgical guides, and rehab resources, but Can't Bend? Can't Snap? Can't Stop Laughing! is his most personal and practical endeavor yet. Inspired by conversations with patients, providers, and caregivers, Jason blends deep research with relatable storytelling, heartfelt humor, and the kind of blunt honesty you only get in recovery rooms or physical therapy waiting areas.

Jason believes that healing starts with knowledge, comfort, and a few good laughs. He's passionate about empowering people to advocate for themselves, ask better questions, and take ownership of their recovery—even when that means adjusting expectations and redefining what "normal" looks like.

When he's not writing or interviewing experts, Jason can usually be found testing out the limits of his own joints, reading rehab journals for fun (yes, really), and marveling at how many opinions there are about crutches on the internet.

Packing Tips, Mental Prep, and All the Weird Stuff Nobody Told You About

Can't Bend? Can't Snap? Can't Stop Laughing!

Printed in Dunstable, United Kingdom